DELMAR'S PHYSICAL ASSESSMENT SKILLS

DELMAR'S
PHYSICAL ASSESSMENT
SKILLS

Gaylene Bouska Altman
RN, PhD
Director
Learning Lab
Faculty
School of Nursing
University of Washington
Seattle, Washington

THOMSON
DELMAR LEARNING

Australia Canada Mexico Singapore Spain United Kingdom United States

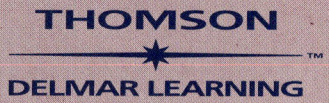

Delmar's Physical Assessment Skills
Gaylene Bouska Altman

Executive Director, Health Care:
William Brottmiller

Executive Editor:
Cathy L. Esperti

Acquisitions Editor:
Matthew Filimonov

Developmental Editor:
Patricia A. Gaworecki

Executive Marketing Manager:
Dawn F. Gerrain

Channel Manager:
Jennifer McAvey

Editorial Assistant:
Patricia Osborn

Art/Design Coordinator:
Robert Plante

Project Editor:
Mary Ellen Cox

Production Coordinator:
Catherine Ciardullo

Technology Project Manager:
Laurie Davis

COPYRIGHT © 2004 by Delmar Learning, a division of Thomson Learning, Inc. Thomson Learning™ is a trademark used herein under license.

Printed in the United States of America
1 2 3 4 5 XXX 07 06 05 04 03 02

For more information, contact Delmar Learning, 5 Maxwell Drive, Clifton Park, NY 12065.
Or, find us on the World Wide Web at http://www.delmarhealthcare.com

ALL RIGHTS RESERVED. No part of this work covered by the copyright hereon may be reproduced or used in any form or by any means—graphic, electronic, or mechanical, including photocopying, recording, taping, Web distribution or information storage and retrieval systems—without written permission from the publisher.

For permission to use material from this text or product, contact us by
Tel   (800) 730-2214
Fax (800) 730-2215
www.thomsonrights.com

Library of Congress Cataloging-in-Publication Data:

Altman, Gaylene
  Delmar's physical assessment skills/Gaylene Bouska Altman
      p. cm.
  Includes bibliographical references and index.
  ISBN 1-40182-748-9 (alk. paper)
  1. Nursing assessment. 2. Physical diagnosis. 3. Nursing.
  I. Title: Physical assessment skills. II. Title.

RT48 A45 2002
616.07'5–dc21   2002041122

NOTICE TO THE READER

Publisher does not warrant or guarantee any of the products described herein or perform any independent analysis in connection with any of the product information contained herein. Publisher does not assume, and expressly disclaims, any obligation to obtain and include information other than that provided to it by the manufacturer.

The reader is expressly warned to consider and adopt all safety precautions that might be indicated by the activities herein and to avoid all potential hazards. By following the instructions contained herein, the reader willingly assumes all risks in connection with such instructions.

The publisher makes no representations or warranties of any kind, including but not limited to, the warranties of fitness for particular purpose or merchantability, nor are any such representations implied with respect to the material set forth herein, and the publisher takes no responsibility with respect to such material. The publisher shall not be liable for any special, consequential, or exemplary damages resulting, in whole or part, from the readers' use of, or reliance upon, this material.

Dedication

Dr. Altman would like to dedicate this book and express a special thanks to her husband, Len, and her three children, Jonathan, Matthew, and especially Katherine, who exhibited patience and understanding during this project, and to all the staff and clients at the numerous health facilities who made this book possible. Furthermore, Dr. Altman would like to dedicate this book to professional nurses, health care providers, clients, and families who will benefit from the application of knowledge presented in this publication.

Contents

Multimedia Index		x
Contributors		xvii
Reviewers		xix
Preface		xx
Acknowledgments		xxvi
About the Author		xxvii
References		xxviii

CHAPTER 1 • PHYSICAL ASSESSMENT   1

1-1	Physical Assessment	2
1-2	Taking a Temperature	29
1-3	Taking a Pulse	43
1-4	Counting Respirations	52
1-5	Taking a Blood Pressure	58
1-6	Weighing a Client, Mobile and Immobile	67
1-7	Measuring Intake and Output	74
1-8	Breast Self-Examination	81
1-9	Male Genitalia, Hernia and Rectal Examination	90
1-10	Collecting a Clean-Catch, Midstream Urine Specimen	99
1-11	Testing Urine for Specific Gravity, Ketones, Glucose, and Occult Blood	106
1-12	Performing a Skin Puncture	114
1-13	Measuring Blood Glucose Levels	120
1-14	Collecting Nose, Throat, and Sputum Specimens	128
1-15	Testing for Occult Blood with a Hemoccult Slide	137

CHAPTER 2 • SAFETY AND INFECTION CONTROL   XXX

2-1	Proper Body Mechanics and Safe Lifting/Transferring	XX
2-2	Assisting with Ambulation and Safe Falling	XX
2-3	Applying Restraints	XXX
2-4	Hand Washing	XX
2-5	Donning and Removing Clean and Contaminated Gloves, Cap, and Mask	XXX
2-6	Removing Contaminated Items	XXX
2-7	Applying Sterile Gloves via the Open Method	XXX
2-8	Surgical Scrub	XXX
2-9	Applying Sterile Gloves and Gown via the Closed Method	XXX
2-10	Emergency Airway Management	XXX
2-11	Administering Cardiopulmonary Resuscitation (CPR)	XXX
2-12	Performing the Heimlich Maneuver	XXX
2-13	Responding to Accidental Poisoning	XXX
2-14	Emergency Client Transport	XXX

CHAPTER 3 • PATIENT CARE AND COMFORT   XXX

3-1	The Effective Communication Process	XXX
3-2	Guided Imagery	XXX
3-3	Progressive Muscle Relaxation	XXX
3-4	Therapeutic Massage	XXX
3-5	Applying Moist Heat	XXX
3-6	Warm Soaks and Sitz Baths	XXX
3-7	Applying Dry Heat	XXX
3-8	Using a Thermal Blanket and an Infant Radiant Heat Warmer	XXX
3-9	Applying Cold Treatment	XXX
3-10	Assisting with a Transcutaneous Electrical Nerve Stimulation (TENS) Unit	XXX

CHAPTER 4 • BASIC CARE   XXX

4-1	Changing Linens in an Unoccupied Bed	XXX
4-2	Changing Linens in an Occupied Bed	XXX
4-3	Turning and Positioning a Client	XXX
4-4	Moving a Client in Bed	XXX
4-5	Assisting with a Bedpan or Urinal	XXX

4-6	Assisting with Feeding	XXX
4-7	Bathing a Client in Bed	XXX
4-8	Oral Care	XXX
4-9	Perineal and Genital Care	XXX
4-10	Eye Care	XXX
4-11	Hair and Scalp Care	XXX
4-12	Hand and Foot Care	XXX
4-13	Shaving a Client	XXX
4-14	Giving a Back Rub	XXX
4-15	Changing the IV Gown	XXX
4-16	Assisting from Bed to Stretcher	XXX
4-17	Assisting from Bed to Wheelchair, Commode, or Chair	XXX
4-18	Assisting from Bed to Walking	XXX
4-19	Using a Hydraulic Lift	XXX
4-20	Administering Preoperative Care	XXX
4-21	Preparing a Surgical Site	XXX
4-22	Assessing Immediate Postoperative Care	XXX
4-23	Postoperative Exercise Instruction	XXX
4-24	Administering Passive Range of Motion (ROM) Exercises	XXX
4-25	Postmortem Care	XXX

CHAPTER 5 • MEDICATION ADMINISTRATION XXX

5-1	Administering Oral, Sublingual, and Buccal Medications	XXX
5-2	Administering Eye and Ear Medications	XXX
5-3	Administering Skin/Topical Medications	XXX
5-4	Administering Nasal Medications	XXX
5-5	Administering Rectal Medications	XXX
5-6	Administering Vaginal Medications	XXX
5-7	Administering Nebulized Medications	XXX
5-8	Administering an Intradermal Injection	XXX
5-9	Administering a Subcutaneous Injection	XXX
5-10	Administering an Intramuscular Injection	XXX
5-11	Administering Medication via Z-track Injection	XXX
5-12	Withdrawing Medication from a Vial	XXX
5-13	Withdrawing Medication from an Ampoule	XXX
5-14	Mixing Medications from Two Vials into One Syringe	XXX
5-15	Preparing an IV Solution	XXX
5-16	Adding Medications to an IV Solution	XXX
5-17	Administering Medications via Secondary Administration Sets (Piggyback)	XXX
5-18	Administering Medications via IV Bolus or IV Push	XXX
5-19	Administering Medications via Volume-Control Sets	XXX
5-20	Administering Medication via a Cartridge System	XXX
5-21	Administering Patient-Controlled Analgesia (PCA)	XXX
5-22	Administering Epidural Analgesia	XXX
5-23	Managing Controlled Substances	XXX

CHAPTER 6 • NUTRITION AND ELIMINATION XXX

6-1	Inserting and Maintaining a Nasogastric Tube	XXX
6-2	Assessing Placement of a Large-Bore Feeding Tube	XXX
6-3	Assessing Placement of a Small-Bore Feeding Tube	XXX
6-4	Removing a Nasogastric Tube	XXX
6-5	Feeding and Medicating via a Gastrostomy Tube	XXX
6-6	Maintaining Gastrointestinal Suction Devices	XXX
6-7	Applying a Condom Catheter	XXX
6-8	Inserting an Indwelling Catheter: Male	XXX
6-9	Inserting an Indwelling Catheter: Female	XXX
6-10	Routine Catheter Care	XXX
6-11	Obtaining a Residual Urine Specimen from an Indwelling Catheter	XXX
6-12	Irrigating a Urinary Catheter	XXX
6-13	Irrigating the Bladder Using a Closed-System Catheter	XXX
6-14	Removing an Indwelling Catheter	XXX
6-15	Catheterizing a Noncontinent Urinary Diversion	XXX

6-16	Maintaining a Continent Urinary Diversion	XXX
6-17	Pouching a Noncontinent Urinary Diversion	XXX
6-18	Administering Peritoneal Dialysis	XXX
6-19	Administering an Enema	XXX
6-20	Digital Removal of Fecal Impaction	XXX
6-21	Inserting a Rectal Tube	XXX
6-22	Irrigating and Cleaning a Stoma	XXX
6-23	Changing a Bowel Diversion Ostomy Appliance: Pouching a Stoma	XXX

CHAPTER 7 • OXYGENATION   XXX

7-1	Administering Oxygen Therapy	XXX
7-2	Assisting a Client with Controlled Coughing and Deep Breathing	XXX
7-3	Assisting a Client with an Incentive Spirometer	XXX
7-4	Administering Pulmonary Therapy and Postural Drainage	XXX
7-5	Administering Pulse Oximetry	XXX
7-6	Measuring Peak Expiratory Flow Rates	XXX
7-7	Administering Intermittent Positive-Pressure Breathing (IPPB)	XXX
7-8	Assisting with Continuous Positive Airway Pressure (CPAP)	XXX
7-9	Preparing the Chest Drainage System	XXX
7-10	Maintaining the Chest Tube and Chest Drainage System	XXX
7-11	Measuring the Output from a Chest Drainage System	XXX
7-12	Obtaining a Specimen from a Chest Drainage System	XXX
7-13	Removing a Chest Tube	XXX
7-14	Ventilating the Client with an Ambu Bag	XXX
7-15	Inserting the Pharyngeal Airway	XXX
7-16	Maintaining Mechanical Ventilation	XXX
7-17	Suctioning Endotracheal and Tracheal Tubes	XXX
7-18	Maintaining and Cleaning Endotracheal Tubes	XXX
7-19	Maintaining and Cleaning the Tracheostomy Tube	XXX
7-20	Maintaining a Double Cannula Tracheostomy Tube	XXX
7-21	Plugging the Tracheostomy Tube	XXX

CHAPTER 8 • CIRCULATORY   XXX

8-1	Performing Venipuncture (Blood Drawing)	XXX
8-2	Starting an IV	XXX
8-3	Inserting a Butterfly Needle	XXX
8-4	Preparing the IV Bag and Tubing	XXX
8-5	Setting the IV Flow Rate	XXX
8-6	Assessing and Maintaining an IV Insertion Site	XXX
8-7	Changing the IV Solution	XXX
8-8	Discontinuing the IV and Changing to a Saline Lock	XXX
8-9	Administering a Blood Transfusion	XXX
8-10	Assessing and Responding to Transfusion Reactions	XXX
8-11	Assisting with the Insertion of a Central Venous Catheter	XXX
8-12	Changing the Central Venous Dressing	XXX
8-13	Changing the Central Venous Tubing	XXX
8-14	Maintaining a Central Venous Catheter	XXX
8-15	Measuring Central Venous Pressure (CVP)	XXX
8-16	Drawing Blood from a Central Venous Catheter	XXX
8-17	Infusing Total Parenteral Nutrition (TPN) and Fat Emulsion through a Central Venous Catheter	XXX
8-18	Removing the Central Venous Catheter	XXX
8-19	Inserting a Peripherally Inserted Central Catheter (PICC)	XXX
8-20	Administering Peripheral Vein Total Parenteral Nutrition	XXX
8-21	Hemodialysis Site Care	XXX
8-22	Using an Implantable Venous Access Device	XXX
8-23	Caring for an Implanted Venous Access Device	XXX
8-24	Obtaining an Arterial Blood Gas Specimen	XXX
8-25	Assisting with the Insertion and Maintenance of an Epidural Catheter	XXX

CHAPTER 9 • SKIN INTEGRITY AND WOUND CARE   XXX

9-1	Bandaging	XXX
9-2	Applying a Dry Dressing	XXX

9-3	Applying a Wet-to-Damp Dressing (Wet-to-Dry-to-Moist Dressing)	XXX	10-9	External Fixation or Skeletal Traction Pin Care	XXX
9-4	Applying a Transparent Dressing	XXX	10-10	Assisting with Casting—Plaster and Fiberglass	XXX
9-5	Applying a Pressure Bandage	XXX	10-11	Cast Care and Comfort	XXX
9-6	Changing Dressings around Therapeutic Puncture Sites	XXX	10-12	Cast Bivalving and Windowing	XXX
9-7	Irrigating a Wound	XXX	10-13	Cast Removal	XXX
9-8	Packing a Wound	XXX	10-14	Assisting with a Continuous Passive Motion Device	XXX
9-9	Cleaning and Dressing a Wound with an Open Drain	XXX	10-15	Assisting with Crutches, Cane, or Walker	XXX
9-10	Dressing a Wound with Retention Sutures	XXX			

CHAPTER 11 • SPECIAL PROCEDURES XXX

9-11	Obtaining a Wound Drainage Specimen for Culturing	XXX
9-12	Maintaining a Closed Wound Drainage System	XXX
9-13	Care of the Jackson-Pratt (JP) Drain Site and Emptying the Drain Bulb	XXX
9-14	Removing Skin Sutures and Staples	XXX
9-15	Preventing and Managing the Pressure Ulcer	XXX
9-16	Managing Irritated Peristomal Skin	XXX
9-17	Pouching a Draining Wound	XXX

11-1	Administering an Electrocardiogram	XXX
11-2	Magnetic Resonance Imaging (MRI)	XXX
11-3	Assisting with Computed Tomography (CT) Scanning	XXX
11-4	Assisting with a Liver Biopsy	XXX
11-5	Assisting with a Thoracentesis	XXX
11-6	Assisting with Abdominal Paracentesis	XXX
11-7	Assisting with a Bone Marrow Biopsy/Aspiration	XXX
11-8	Assisting with a Lumbar Puncture	XXX
11-9	Assisting with Amniocentesis	XXX
11-10	Assisting with Bronchoscopy	XXX
11-11	Assisting with Gastrointestinal Endoscopy	XXX
11-12	Assisting with a Proctosigmoidoscopy	XXX
11-13	Assisting with Arteriography	XXX
11-14	Positron-Emission Tomography Scanning	XXX

CHAPTER 10 • IMMOBILIZATION AND SUPPORT XXX

10-1	Applying an Elastic Bandage	XXX
10-2	Applying a Splint	XXX
10-3	Applying an Arm Sling	XXX
10-4	Applying Antiembolic Stockings	XXX
10-5	Applying a Pneumatic Compression Device	XXX
10-6	Applying Abdominal, T-, or Breast Binders	XXX
10-7	Applying Skin Traction—Adhesive and Nonadhesive	XXX
10-8	Maintaining and Monitoring Skeletal Traction	XXX

REFERENCES XXX

INDEX XXX

Multimedia Index

The reference and learning value of this skills book is enhanced by its multimedia companion pieces. First, each of the skills in this book is presented in a rich, multimedia environment that enables users to review and learn vital nursing skills on an independent basis. Additionally, over 100 of the skills have engaging step-by-step 5-10 minute video presentations that aid in comprehension and implementation of key actions and rationales. Over 1500 full color, real-life photographs further enhance learning. Next, an accompanying video series clearly demonstrates over 100 of the skills contained within the second edition of Delmar's *Fundamental & Advanced Nursing Skills* in concise 5-10 minute presentations. These video segments carefully show users step-by-step actions and reinforce learning. These rich multimedia companions supplement and reinforce the content found within Delmar's *Fundamental & Advanced Nursing Skills,* second edition.

The following table indicates in which DVD-ROM or video set a particular skill may be found. An AC, BC, or IC, indicates that the skill may be found on the corresponding advanced, basic, or intermediate skills DVD-ROM. The last column of the table indicates the location of each skill on VHS video tape.

CHAPTER 1 • PHYSICAL ASSESSMENT

SKILL	SKILL TITLE	PAGE	DVD	TAPE
1-1	Physical assessment	2	BC	1
1-2	Taking a temperature	28	BC	2
1-3	Taking a pulse	40	BC	2
1-4	Counting respirations	47	BC	2
1-5	Taking blood pressure	53	BC	2
1-6	Weighing a client, mobile and immobile	61	BC	2
1-7	Measuring intake and output	68	IC	7
1-8	Breast examination	74	BC	
1-9	Male genitalia, hernia, and rectal examination	74	BC	
1-10	Collecting a clean-catch, midstream urine specimen	82	IC	7
1-11	Testing urine for specific gravity, ketones, and occult blood	89	BC	
1-12	Performing a skin puncture	96	IC	7
1-13	Measuring blood glucose levels	101	BC	
1-14	Collecting nose, throat, and sputum specimens	108	IC	7
1-15	Testing for occult blood with a hemoccult slide	116	BC	

CHAPTER 2 • SAFETY AND INFECTION CONTROL

2-1	Proper body mechanics and safe lifting/transferring	XXX	BC	

MULTIMEDIA INDEX

SKILL	SKILL TITLE	PAGE	DVD	TAPE
2-2	Assisting with ambulation and safe falling	XXX	BC	
2-3	Applying Restraints	XXX	BC	4
2-4	Hand Washing	XXX	BC	5
2-5	Donning and removing clean and contaminated gloves, cap, and mask	XXX	BC	
2-6	Removing contaminated items	XXX	BC	
2-7	Applying sterile gloves via the open method	XXX	BC	
2-8	Surgical Scrub	XXX	BC	
2-9	Applying sterile gloves and gown via the closed method	XXX	BC	
2-10	Emergency airway management	XXX	BC	
2-11	Administering cardiopulmonary resuscitation (CPR)	XXX	BC	
2-12	Performing the Heimlich maneuver	XXX	BC	
2-13	Responding to accidental poisoning	XXX	BC	
2-14	Emergency client transport	XXX	BC	

CHAPTER 3 • PATIENT CARE AND COMFORT

SKILL	SKILL TITLE	PAGE	DVD	TAPE
3-1	The effective communication process	XXX	BC	
3-2	Guided imagery	XXX	BC	
3-3	Progressive muscle relaxation	XXX	BC	
3-4	Therapeutic Massage	XXX	BC	
3-5	Applying moist heat	XXX	BC	
3-6	Warm soaks and sitz baths	XXX	BC	
3-7	Applying dry heat	XXX	BC	
3-8	Using a thermal blanket and an infant radiant heat warmer	XXX	BC	
3-9	Applying cold treatment	XXX	BC	
3-10	Assisting with a transcutaneous electrical nerve stimulator (TENS) unit	XXX	BC	

CHAPTER 4 • BASIC CARE

SKILL	SKILL TITLE	PAGE	DVD	TAPE
4-1	Changing linens in an unoccupied bed	XXX	BC	4
4-2	Changing linens in an occupied bed	XXX	BC	4
4-3	Turning and positioning a client	XXX	BC	6
4-4	Moving a client in bed	XXX	BC	6
4-5	Assisting with a bedpan or urinal	XXX	BC	
4-6	Assisting with feeding	XXX	BC	
4-7	Bathing a patient in bed	XXX	BC	5
4-8	Oral care	XXX	BC	3
4-9	Perineal and genital care	XXX	BC	5
4-10	Eye care	XXX	BC	3
4-11	Hair and scalp care	XXX	BC	3

MULTIMEDIA INDEX

SKILL	SKILL TITLE	PAGE	DVD	TAPE
4-12	Hand and foot care	XXX	BC	3
4-13	Shaving a client	XXX	BC	3
4-14	Giving a back rub	XXX	BC	5
4-15	Changing the IV gown	XXX	BC	
4-16	Assisting from bed to stretcher	XXX	BC	6
4-17	Assisting from bed to wheelchair, commode, or chair	XXX	BC	6
4-18	Assisting from bed to walking	XXX	BC	6
4-19	Using a hydraulic lift	XXX	BC	
4-20	Administering preoperative care	XXX	BC	
4-21	Preparing a surgical site	XXX	BC	
4-22	Administering immediate postoperative care	XXX	BC	
4-23	Postoperative exercise instruction	XXX	BC	
4-24	Administering passive range of motion (ROM) exercises	XXX	BC	6
4-25	Postmortem care	XXX	BC	

CHAPTER 5 • MEDICATION ADMINISTRATION

SKILL	SKILL TITLE	PAGE	DVD	TAPE
5-1	Administering oral, sublingual, and buccal medications	XXX	AC	14
5-2	Administering eye and ear medications	XXX	AC	14
5-3	Administering skin/topical medications	XXX	AC	14
5-4	Administering nasal medications	XXX	AC	14
5-5	Administering rectal medications	XXX	AC	14
5-6	Administering vaginal medications	XXX	AC	14
5-7	Administering nebulized medications	XXX	AC	14
5-8	Administering an intradermal injection	XXX	AC	15
5-9	Administering a subcutaneous injection	XXX	AC	15
5-10	Administering an intramuscular injection	XXX	AC	15
5-11	Administering medication via Z-track injection	XXX	AC	15
5-12	Withdrawing medication from a vial	XXX	AC	15
5-13	Withdrawing medication from an ampoule	XXX	AC	15
5-14	Mixing medications from two vials into one syringe	XXX	AC	15
5-15	Preparing an IV solution	XXX	AC	16
5-16	Adding medications to an IV solution	XXX	AC	16
5-17	Administering medications via secondary administration sets (piggyback)	XXX	AC	16

MULTIMEDIA INDEX

SKILL	SKILL TITLE	PAGE	DVD	TAPE
5-18	Administering medications via IV bolus or IV push	XXX	AC	16
5-19	Administering medications via volume-control sets	XXX	AC	16
5-20	Administering medication via a cartridge system	XXX	AC	16
5-21	Administering patient-controlled analgesia (PCA)	XXX	AC	16
5-22	Administering epidural analgesia	XXX	AC	
5-23	Managing controlled substances	XXX	AC	13

CHAPTER 6 • NUTRITION AND ELIMINATION

SKILL	SKILL TITLE	PAGE	DVD	TAPE
6-1	Inserting and maintaining a nasogastric tube	XXX	IC	8
6-2	Assessing placement of a large-bore feeding tube	XXX	IC	12
6-3	Assessing placement of a small-bore feeding tube	XXX	IC	8
6-4	Removing a nasogastric tube	XXX	IC	8
6-5	Feeding and medicating via a gastrostomy tube	XXX	IC	8
6-6	Maintaining gastrointestinal suction devices	XXX	IC	8
6-7	Applying a condom catheter	XXX	IC	9
6-8	Inserting an indwelling catheter: male	XXX	IC	9
6-9	Inserting an indwelling catheter: female	XXX	IC	9
6-10	Routine catheter care	XXX	IC	9
6-11	Obtaining a residual urine specimen from an indwelling catheter	XXX	IC	7
6-12	Irrigating a urinary catheter	XXX	IC	9
6-13	Irrigating the bladder using a closed-system catheter	XXX	IC	
6-14	Removing an indwelling catheter	XXX	IC	
6-15	Catheterizing a noncontinent urinary diversion	XXX	IC	
6-16	Maintaining a continent urinary diversion	XXX	IC	
6-17	Pouching a noncontinent urinary diversion	XXX	IC	
6-18	Administering peritoneal dialysis	XXX	IC	
6-19	Administering an enema	XXX	IC	10
6-20	Digital removal of fecal impaction	XXX	IC	10
6-21	Inserting a rectal tube	XXX	IC	10
6-22	Irrigating and cleaning a stoma	XXX	IC	10
6-23	Changing a bowel diversion ostomy appliance–pouching a stoma	XXX	IC	10

SKILL	SKILL TITLE	PAGE	DVD	TAPE
CHAPTER 7 • OXYGENATION				
7-01	Administering oxygen therapy	XXX	AC	20
7-02	Assisting a client with controlled coughing and deep breathing	XXX	AC	20
7-03	Assisting a client with an incentive spirometer	XXX	AC	
7-04	Administering pulmonary therapy and postural drainage	XXX	AC	
7-05	Administering pulse oximetry	XXX	AC	
7-06	Measuring peak expiratory flow rates	XXX	AC	20
7-07	Administering intermittent positive-pressure breathing (IPPB)	XXX	AC	
7-08	Assisting with continuous positive airway pressure (CPAP)	XXX	AC	
7-09	Preparing the chest drainage system	XXX	AC	
7-10	Maintaining the chest tube and chest drainage system	XXX	AC	
7-11	Measuring the output from a chest drainage system	XXX	AC	
7-12	Obtaining a specimen from a chest drainage system	XXX	AC	
7-13	Removing a chest tube	XXX	AC	
7-14	Ventilating the patient with an ambu bag	XXX	AC	
7-15	Inserting the pharyngeal airway	XXX	AC	
7-16	Maintaining mechanical ventilation	XXX	AC	
7-17	Suctioning endotracheal and tracheal tubes	XXX	AC	
7-18	Maintaining and cleaning endotracheal tubes	XXX	AC	
7-19	Maintaining and cleaning the tracheostomy tube	XXX	AC	
7-20	Maintaining a double cannula tracheostomy tube	XXX	AC	
7-21	Plugging the tracheostomy tube	XXX	AC	
CHAPTER 8 • CIRCULATORY				
8-01	Performing venipuncture (Blood Drawing)	XXX	AC	17
8-02	Starting an IV	XXX	AC	17
8-03	Inserting a butterfly needle	XXX	AC	17
8-04	Preparing the IV bag and tubing	XXX	AC	17
8-05	Setting the IV flow rate	XXX	AC	18
8-06	Assessing and maintaining an IV insertion site	XXX	AC	18
8-07	Changing the IV solution	XXX	AC	18

MULTIMEDIA INDEX

SKILL	SKILL TITLE	PAGE	DVD	TAPE
8-08	Discontinuing the IV and changing to a saline lock	XXX	AC	18
8-09	Administering a blood transfusion	XXX	AC	19
8-10	Assessing and responding to transfusion reactions	XXX	AC	19
8-11	Assisting with the insertion of a central venous catheter	XXX	IC	
8-12	Changing the central venous dressing	XXX	IC	
8-13	Changing the central venous tubing	XXX	IC	
8-14	Flushing a central venous catheter	XXX	IC	
8-15	Measuring central venous pressure (CVP)	XXX	IC	
8-16	Drawing blood from a central venous catheter	XXX	IC	
8-17	Infusing total parenteral nutrition (TPN) and fat emulsion through a central venous catheter	XXX	IC	
8-18	Removing the central venous catheter	XXX	IC	
8-19	Inserting a peripherally inserted central catheter (PICC)	XXX	IC	
8-20	Administering peripheral vein total parenteral nutrition	XXX	IC	
8-21	Hemodialysis site care	XXX	IC	
8-22	Using an implantable venous access device	XXX	IC	
8-23	Caring for an implanted venous access device	XXX	IC	
8-24	Obtaining an arterial blood gas specimen	XXX	IC	
8-25	Assisting with the insertion and maintaining an epidural catheter	XXX	IC	

CHAPTER 9 • SKIN INTEGRITY AND WOUND CARE

SKILL	SKILL TITLE	PAGE	DVD	TAPE
9-01	Bandaging	XXX	IC	11
9-02	Applying a dry dressing	XXX	IC	11
9-03	Applying a wet-to-damp dressing (wet-to-dry-to-moist dressing)	XXX	IC	11
9-04	Applying a transparent dressing	XXX	IC	11
9-05	Applying a pressure bandage	XXX	IC	11
9-06	Changing dressings around therapeutic puncture sites	XXX	IC	11
9-07	Irrigating a wound	XXX	IC	12
9-08	Packing a wound	XXX	IC	12
9-09	Cleaning and dressing a wound with an open drain	XXX	IC	12
9-10	Dressing a wound with retention sutures	XXX	IC	12
9-11	Obtaining a wound drainage specimen for culturing	XXX	IC	7
9-12	Maintaining a closed wound drainage system	XXX	IC	12

SKILL	SKILL TITLE	PAGE	DVD	TAPE
9-13	Care of the Jackson-Pratt (JP) drain site and emptying the drain bulb	XXX	IC	
9-14	Removing skin sutures and staples	XXX	IC	12
9-15	Preventing and managing the pressure ulcer	XXX	BC	6
9-16	Managing irritated peristomal skin	XXX	IC	
9-17	Pouching a draining wound	XXX	IC	12

CHAPTER 10 • IMMOBILIZATION AND SUPPORT

SKILL	SKILL TITLE	PAGE	DVD	TAPE
10-01	Applying an elastic bandage	XXX	BC	
10-02	Applying a splint	XXX	BC	
10-03	Applying an arm sling	XXX	BC	
10-04	Applying antiembolic stockings	XXX	BC	
10-05	Applying a pneumatic compression device	XXX	BC	
10-06	Applying abdominal, T-, or breast binders	XXX	BC	
10-07	Applying skin traction-adhesive and nonadhesive	XXX	BC	
10-08	Maintaining and monitoring skeletal traction	XXX	BC	
10-09	External fixation or skeletal traction pin care	XXX	BC	
10-10	Assisting with casting – plaster and fiberglass	XXX	BC	
10-11	Cast care and comfort	XXX	BC	
10-12	Cast bivalving and windowing	XXX	BC	
10-13	Cast removal	XXX	BC	
10-14	Assisting with a continuous passive motion device	XXX	BC	
10-15	Assisting with crutches, cane, or walker	XXX	BC	

CHAPTER 11 • SPECIAL PROCEDURES

SKILL	SKILL TITLE	PAGE	DVD	TAPE
11-01	Administering an electrocardiogram	XXX	AC	
11-02	Magnetic Resonance Imaging (MRI)	XXX	AC	
11-03	Assisting with computed tomography (CT) scanning	XXX	AC	
11-04	Assisting with a liver biopsy	XXX	AC	
11-05	Assisting with a thoracentesis	XXX	AC	
11-06	Assisting with an abdominal paracentesis	XXX	AC	
11-07	Assisting with a bone marrow biopsy/aspiration	XXX	AC	
11-08	Assisting with a lumbar puncture	XXX	AC	
11-09	Assisting with amniocentesis	XXX	AC	
11-10	Assisting with bronchoscopy	XXX	AC	
11-11	Assisting with a gastrointestinal endoscopy	XXX	AC	
11-12	Assisting with a proctosigmoidoscopy	XXX	AC	
11-13	Assisting with arteriography	XXX	AC	
11-14	Positron-emission tomography scanning	XXX	AC	

Contributors

Patricia Abott, RN, MSN, ARNP
University of Washington Medical Center
School of Nursing, University of Washington
Seattle, WA

Sharon Aronovitch, RN, PhD, CETN
Regents College
Albany, NY

Dale D. Barb, MHS, PT
Academic Coordinator of Clinical Education
Department of Physical Therapy
Wichita State University
Wichita, KS

Susan Weiss Behrend, RN, MSN
Fox Chase Cancer Center
Philadelphia, PA

Bethaney Campbell, RN, MN, OCN
University of Washington Medical Center
Seattle, WA

Curt Campbell
Integrated Health Services of Seattle
Seattle, WA

Nancy Chambers, RN, BSN
University of Washington Medical Center
Seattle, WA

Jung-Chen (Kristina) Chang, RN, MN
University of Washington
School of Nursing
Seattle, WA

Eileen M. Collins, RN, MN, ARNP
School of Nursing
University of Washington
Seattle, WA

Cheryl L. Cooke, RN, MN
Student Services Coordinator
University of Washington
School of Nursing
Seattle, WA

Gayle C. Crawford, RN, BSN
Staff Nurse
University of Washington Medical Center
Seattle, WA

Mary Doyle, RN, MS
Maria College, Nursing Faculty
Niskayuna, NY

Eleonor U. de la Pena, BS
Northwest Asthma and Allergy Center
Seattle, WA

Jeanne Erickson, RN, MSN, AOCN
University of Virginia Cancer Center
Portsmouth, VA

Tom Ewing, RN, BSN
Hematology-Oncology
University of Washington Medical Center
Seattle, WA

Stacy Frish, RN, BSN
University of Washington Medical Center
Seattle, WA

Eva Gallagher, RN, BSN
Methodist Hospital
Minneapolis, MN

Susan Boyce Gilmore, MN, RN, CCRN
Lecturer, Biobehavior Nursing and Health Systems
University of Washington
School of Nursing
Seattle, WA

Hsiu-Ying Huang, RN, PhD
University of Washington
School of Nursing
Seattle, WA

Kimberly Hudson, RN, MN
University of Washington Medical Center
Seattle, WA

CONTRIBUTORS

Karrin Johnson, RN
Health Care Project Manager
NRSPACE Software, Inc.
Bellevue, WA

Kimberly Sue Kahn, RN, MSN, FNP, AOCN
University of Virginia
Portsmouth, VA

Catherine H. Kelley, RN, MSN, OCN
Chimeric Therapies, Inc.
Palatine, IL

Carla A. Bouska Lee, PhD, ARNP, FAAN
Clarkston College
Omaha, NE

Kathryn Lilleby, RN
Clinical Research Nurse
Fred Hutchinson Cancer Research Center
Seattle, WA

Joan M. Mack, RN, MSN
Nebraska Medical Center
Omaha, NE

Patricia McDowell, RPPT
University of Washington Medical Center
Seattle, WA

Peter C. Meyer, RRT
University of Washington Medical Center
Seattle, WA

Marianne Frances Moore, RN, MSN
Clarkson Hospital
Omaha, NE

Agnes Morrison, RN, MSN
Department of Nursing
Thomas Jefferson University
Philadelphia, PA

Claretta D. Munger, MSN, ARNP
Newman Grove, NE

Susan Randolph, RN, MSN
Manager, Transplant Services
Coram Healthcare
Parkerburg, WV

Sally Ann Rinehart, RN, BSN
Nursing Lab Supervisor
Pacific Lutheran University
Tacoma, WA

Susan Rives, RN, BSN, OCN
CARE Center Coordinator
Martha Jefferson Hospital
Charlottesville, VA

Barbara Sigler, RN, MNEd, CORLN
Technical Publications Editor
Oncology Nursing Press, Inc.
Formerly: Clinical Nurse Specialist in
Otolaryngology—Head and Neck Surgery
University of Pittsburgh Medical Center
Pittsburgh, PA

Marilyn Stapleton, RNC, MS
Excelsior College
Albany, NY

Pam Talley, RN, PhD
University of Washington
School of Nursing
Seattle, WA

Hsin-Yi (Jean) Tang, RN, MS
School of Nursing
University of Washington
Seattle, WA

Samuel C. Taylor, RN
Assistant Nurse Manager, Orthopedics
Harborview Medical Center
Seattle, WA

Robi Thomas, MS, RN, AOCN
Clinical Nurse Specialist for Oncology
and the Pain Center
St. Mary's Mercy Medical Center
Grand Rapids, MI

Nancy Unger, RN, MN, MPH
University of Washington
Seattle, WA

Chandra VanPaepeghem, RN, BSN
University of Washington Medical Center
Seattle, WA

Debra A. Bovinett Wolf, RN, BSN, MPH
Roosevelt Pain Center
University of Washington Medical Center
Seattle, WA

Reviewers

Marie H. Ahrens, MS, RN: University of Tulsa, Tulsa, OK

Danette Birkhimer, RN, MS, OCN: College of Nursing, Ohio State University, Columbus, OH

Teri Boese, MS, RN: The University of Iowa, Iowa City, IA

Kathy Campbell: Maria College, Albany, NY

Brenda Cherry, RN, MSN, CCRN: DeKalb College, Decatur, GA

Pam Covault, RN, MS: Neosho County Community College, Ottawa, KS

Sandra E. Crowell, MSN, BSN: Wilcox College of Nursing, Middletown, CT

Linda Daley, RN, PhD: College of Nursing, Ohio State University, Columbus, OH

Laura Downes, PhD, MSN, BSN, RN: Springfield Technical Community College, Springfield, MA

Mary C. Doyle, BS, MS, CCRN: Maria College, Troy, NY

Carol Fowler Durham, RN, MSN: University of North Carolina—Chapel Hill, Chapel Hill, NC

Rebecca Gesler, RN, MSN: St. Catharine College, St. Catharine, KY

Deborah J. Gutshall, MSN, CRNP: Harrisburg Area Community College, Harrisburg, PA

Melinda Hamilton, RN, MSN: Pensacola Community College, Pensacola, FL

Cynthia Horvath, RN: Glens Falls Hospital, Glens Falls, NY

Valerie Howard, RN, MS: University of Pittsburg, School of Nursing, Venetia, PA

Bonnie Kirkpatrick, RN, MS, CNS: College of Nursing, Ohio State University, Columbus, OH

Clare Lamontagne, RN, MS: Springfield Technical Community College, Springfield, MA

Verlene Meyer, RN, MN: Walla Walla College, Portland, OR

Mary Moriarty Tarbell, MSN, RN: Springfield Technical Community College, Springfield, MA

Martha Nelson, RN, BSN, CETN, CCM: Florida Community College, University of North Florida, Jacksonville, FL

Joan C. Oliver, EdD, RN: Mt. Hood Community College, Gresham, OR

Marie Ostoyich, RN, MS, CDE: Hudson Valley Community College, Troy, NY

Diana Prouty, RN, MS: St. Luke's College, Kansas City, MO

Diane Sheets, RN, MS: College of Nursing, Ohio State University, Columbus, OH

Martha B. Spear, RN, MSN: Harrisburg Area Community College, Harrisburg, PA

Carol A. Vogt, RN, PhD: Cabarrus College of Health Sciences, Concord, NC

Barbara Voshall, RN, MS: Graceland University, Independence, MO

Preface

Health Care is changing at an increasingly fast pace. The cumulative effects of sophisticated technology, an aging population of clients with chronic disease and long-term sequalae, an increasingly diverse population, and a growing nursing shortage challenge nurses today as never before. Often, nurses are placed in situations that demand an increased level of performance despite a decreased amount of support from the health care system.

Delmar's Fundamental & Advanced Nursing Skills, second edition was revised with this nursing population in mind. This book was developed as a text and guideline to perform the skills used in daily nursing practice, and as a learning tool for new nurses. It was designed to be a usable volume, presenting concepts and actions clearly so that a nurse – whether a novice or an old hand – may retain and master both the skill and the underlying rationale.

The second edition still serves this purpose. Nursing students, registered nurses, licensed practical/vocational nurses, physician assistants, nurse practitioners, certified aids, medical assistants, and any health care worker charged with performing common procedures will value the useful guidelines and principles discussed within this book.

The second edition of *Delmar's Fundamental & Advanced Nursing Skills* addresses the needs of today's changing health care environment by providing nurses and other health care workers with an exciting, new, accompanying video series. Many of the skills within this text are shown in a step-by-step presentation that reinforces the written word. Students and practicing nurses who want to review a nursing procedure may now observe how that skill is carried out by watching a step-by-step video. Over one-hundred skills are presented in video format, and are indicated within the text by use of an icon.

The addition of the accompanying step-by-step videos – each segment between 5 and 10 minutes in length – only enhances the value of this text as a resource to acquire new skills, or as a how-to manual to utilize skills, a procedure manual in a facility, a manual to familiarize a former health care worker reentering health care, or a training manual within a facility. Rather than merely providing a step-by-step implementation, this text may be used to stimulate the reader to learn underlying rationale, analyze expected outcomes of treatment, formulate sound bases for implementation, develop critical thinking skills, and model behavior.

This book contains 203 nursing skills divided into 11 chapters that cover basic and advanced nursing procedures. The practitioner can follow the procedural-manual-type steps presented for each skill to improve competence and comfort levels in performing skills. Standards of nursing practice are maintained in each skill. Research-based knowledge has been incorporated into nursing interventions, especially where controversy may exist.

ORGANIZATION

Each skill is presented using the nursing process: assessment, diagnosis, planning, expected outcomes, implementation, and evaluation. The nursing process is a systematic method whereby nurses can make clinical decisions and delineate a course of action based on analysis of available data. The nursing process is continual and cyclic. Evaluation of the outcome incorporates a feedback loop leading to further assessment, decision making, and implementation of care.

North American Nursing Diagnosis Association (NANDA)

The diagnosis section of the text is based on NANDA's standardized list of nursing diagnoses. Using the input of practicing clinicians, NANDA has developed and refined a standardized list of diagnostic labels for use in the nursing process. Using the standardized list as a guideline, the practitioner interprets the assessment data and derives a diagnosis. The standardized diagnoses help guide client treatment by allowing the practitioner to identify rationales for client care and anticipate potential problems.

PREFACE

DOCUMENTATION AND CHARTING

Documentation provides a legal record of the client's status and the care provided. This record is often used as a means for quality assurance, a utilization review of hospital practices, and statistical analysis of client outcomes in areas of infection control, medical, surgical, and nursing practices. Legal documentation of the client's status and care can be used in a court of law to verify client and health care practices.

Charting includes sheets of fact documentation on forms such as flow sheets, including vital signs, fluid intake and output, intravenous records, medication administration records, assessment checklists, and descriptive information. Charting format varies between facilities. Some examples charting types are the nurse's notes organized around subjectively, objectively, assessment, and planning (SOAP); notes organized around client problems or problem-oriented medical record (OMR); notes organized around body systems (systems charting); or a combinations of formats. The legal requirements for charting are dictated by state laws, professional requirements, the Joint Commission on Accreditation of Healthcare Organizations (JCAHO), and individual facility requirements. Most facilities have committees who approve and delineate guidelines for charting.

Client information should be recorded directly on the chart; thereby, avoiding errors in transferring information. For accuracy, many facilities place daily chart forms at the bedside so information can be recorded promptly. Forms generally include flow sheets, assessments, and medication records of varying complexity. Specialized forms include coma scales, seizure precautions reports, and level of consciousness recording. Care maps and treatment plans for routine specialized care are used when the client is expected to recover in a predictable pattern with expected advances each day. Certain forms, such as consent and insurance forms, must be signed by clients or their legal guardian.

Many hospitals have incorporated computerized charting. Often computers are located in clients' rooms for immediate charting and retrieval of information. Many large facilities have adopted computerized systems for administration and charting of medications, laboratory results, and diagnostic testing. Guidelines and strategies for minimizing the risks of computerized charting are essential. Once computer entries are part of the permanent chart, they cannot be deleted; however, policies exist whereby mistaken entries or incorrect information can be explained.

With standard hard copy documentation, guidelines create consistency between facilities. Some examples of consistency are the use of black ink, correction by drawing a single line through the error to mark it, noting the time of each entry, charting the omission of medications and treatments, and signing entries with initial of first name and complete last name plus title.

CLINICAL PRACTICE GUIDELINES FOR PERFORMING A PROCEDURE

In order to utilize this text to maximize learning, the authors have provided guidelines to follow before beginning the procedure and after the procedure is completed.

Before the Procedure

- Practice the procedure with supervision in a clinical setting.
- Read the client's chart.
- Review the treatment plan or verify orders as necessary.
- Review the procedure.
- Assess the client and determine the appropriateness of the procedure.
- Take into consideration the client's/family's cultural and social background when deciding what to teach and when eliciting feedback.
- Employ the aid of an interpreter if there is a language barrier.
- Use visual aids such as flip charts, models, videos, if available, to explain procedure to client/family.
- If family members are to be involved, plan to instruct when they are present, if possible.
- Client and/or family members should be provided with a written set of instructions to take home with them, if needed.
- Plan the procedure.

After the Procedure

- Assess the client and his/her response to the procedure.
- Document the client's response.
- Change the treatment plan as appropriate.

NEW TO THIS EDITION

Videos

Approximately half of the 203 skills found in the text now have accompanying step-by-step video presentation. This allows readers who want to review a nursing procedure to watch how that skill is carried out by viewing the associated video. These video segments are available in two formats, VHS or DVD, for a school or health care institution interested in purchasing the consolidated series. Refer to the multimedia index in this book for skill location on both VHS and DVD.

Additionally, each skill in the text is marked with a VHS and /or DVD icon for additional reference.

DVD-ROMs

Due to variations in learning styles, all of the content within the text is covered in three DVD-ROMs. This software reviews all of the skills in the book in a friendly multimedia environment. These DVD-ROMs include all of the video content within the scope of the video series.

Delmar's Fundamental and Advanced Nursing Skills Network DVD-ROM

ISBN 1-4018-1077-2

In a skills lab environment, this allows students to review the procedures covered within this text at any networked computer. An assessment feature tracks student performance and reports back to the instructor. All of the step-by-step video treatments of the skills within the book are included with the site-license.

Delmar's Fundamental and Advanced Nursing Skills DVD-ROM 3-PACK

ISBN 1-4018-1075-6

The three-pack DVD-ROM includes all of the DVD-ROMs available to accompany the text. This includes the Basic Care, Intermediate Care, and Advanced Care DVD-ROMs.

Delmar's Basic Care Nursing Skills DVD-ROM

ISBN 1-4018-1071-3

Refer to the multimedia index in this book. Basic skills are identified as BC.

Delmar's Intermediate Nursing Skills DVD-ROM

ISBN 1-4018-1072-1

Refer to the multimedia index in this book. Intermediate skills are marked as IC.

Delmar's Advanced Nursing Care Skills

ISBN 1-4018-1073-X

Refer to the multimedia index in this book. Advanced skills are marked as AC.

Skills

New skills have been added to this edition to clarify essential components of nursing practice. Skill 1-9, Male Genitalia, Hernia, and Rectal Examination was added in response to user feedback to enhance chapter 1, Physical Assessment.

Features

Two new features have been added to the presentation of each nursing procedure. **Delegation Tips**, in a clear, direct manner, provide insights into what a nurse must know about the skill before it is delegated to ancillary personnel. Issues addressed include both technical concerns and legal/ethical aspects of care.

> ▶ **DELEGATION TIPS**
> The skill of respiratory rate measurement is often delegated to ancillary personnel; however, the nurse is responsible for this information and appropriate action. Respiration counts over 30 (adult) or 60 (child) should immediately be reported to the nurse for further assessment.

Special Considerations outline additional factors that may complicate issues or present a special hazard to either a client or nurse. These are issues that the nurse performing a procedure should be mindful of in caring for a client.

> ▶ **SPECIAL CONSIDERATIONS**
> • Never use the thumb to obtain a pulse because you may sense a beat from your own digital artery that can alter an accurate reading.
> • When using a Doppler to obtain a fetal heart beat check the mother's pulse to ensure the beat heard is indeed that of the fetus.
> • When preparing a client for surgery related to venous insufficiency of the lower extremities (i.e., femoral-popliteal bypass), it is essential to mark the pedal pulses with an "X." This facilitates locating the pulse during surgery, to confirm circulation for the surgeon.

SPECIAL FEATURES/UNIQUENESS

Step-by-Step Format. The implementation section is presented in a step-by-step format with rationales for each intervention included. The skill is broken down into simple, easy-to-follow steps with explanations for the underlying reasons for each intervention. This allows even the novice to perform the skill and understand why each step is necessary. The steps presented provide specific directions for performing each skill. However, institutional policies, client condition, environmental setting, and other variables may prompt modification of the interventions presented. When modifications are made, adherence to standards of practice and universal precautions must be maintained. Assess and evaluate the client throughout the procedure, modifying intervention as needed to maintain client safety and security. Rationales provide the scientific basis for each implementation. The rationale enables both the practitioner and client to un-

PREFACE   xxiii

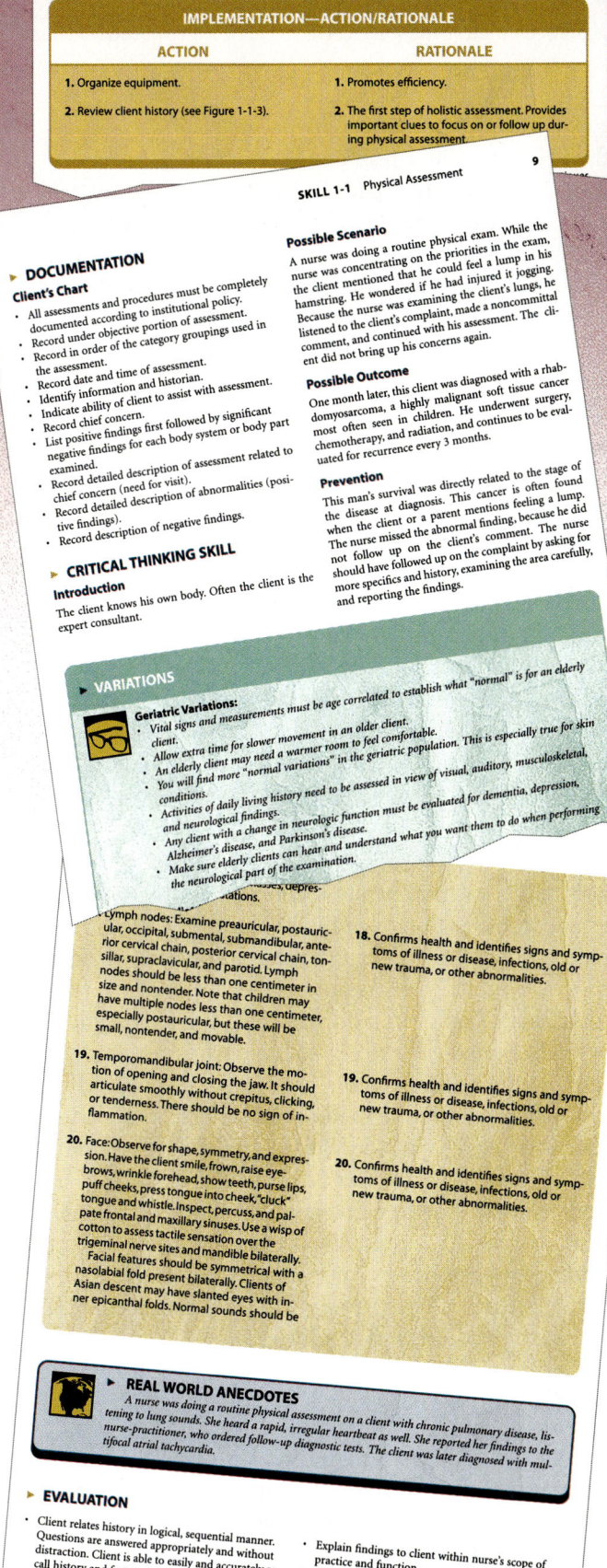

derstand the reason for each implementation, and thus the need to comply with protocols.

Real-life Photographs. The focus of this text is to present reality-based information with photographic examples from current clinical practice, rather than staged or rehearsed scenarios.

Real-world Anecdotes. Client situations drawn from experiences of the contributors or other practitioners add to the immediacy and practicality of the book.

Critical Thinking Skills. This boxed feature offers performance-related scenarios to foster learning, decision making, and analytic thinking. These scenarios often help the reader anticipate possible negative outcomes involved in performing a skill and provide alternatives to avoid unwanted results.

Skill Variations. Variations for each skill are presented for geriatric and pediatric age groups, as well as home-care and long-term care settings, to allow for adaptation of the skills to various situations. For example, geriatric clients may require extra communication skills due to difficulty hearing or understanding. Pediatric clients may need psychosocial assessment of fear or anxiety, or require different sizes of equipment when performing the skill.

Common Errors and Nursing Tips. These are included to assist in improving client outcomes. These sections are presented by experienced nurses to aid and guide the novice practitioner through performing the skills, to help develop competency, and to prevent unwanted outcomes.

Equipment Needed. A list of common equipment needed is provided as an organizational tool to assist in preparation and set-up. The equipment required may vary between institutions.

Estimated Time for Completion. The estimated time to complete a skill is identified to assist in planning and scheduling. The estimated time of completion should be used only as a general guide. Many factors, such as the skill of the practitioner, client cooperation, or degree of client illness, may affect the time required to accomplish a skill.

Client Education Needed. Client teaching should be routinely incorporated when performing skills. Client education is essential in promoting personal health responsibility and compliance. Education should be considered a routine part of most interventions. Informed clients are often less anxious, more cooperative, provide better histories, and are more proactive regarding their health care.

STANDARD PRECAUTIONS

Standard precautions, formerly described as universal precautions, are mandated by either Occupational Safety and Health Administration (OSHA) guidelines or by the Centers for Disease Control (CDC). These are a set of protective guidelines were designed to prevent transmission of any infection, especially bloodborne infections such as human immunodeficiency virus (HIV) and hepatitis B virus (HBV). In general any blood or body fluids are considered potentially infective and direct contact must be avoided. The historical roots of infection control comes from the work of Semmelweis and Lister, but in the United States, the initiation of universal precautions in health care were not in effect until 1985. This came with the increasing awareness of the growing HIV epidemic and the need to protect healthcare workers from exposure to blood and body fluids. The CDC reevaluated universal precautions in 1996 and issued a revised system called standard precautions and transmission-based precautions. Standard precautions are implemented to reduce the risk of transmission of infection from client to healthcare provider and from healthcare provider to client. It incorporates the principles of standard precautions as well as body substance isolation policies and its use is recommended for all hospital clients. Standard precautions apply to blood and all body fluids, secretions and excretions, with the exception of sweat. Body fluids can include cerebrospinal, synovial, pleural, peritoneal, pericardial and amniotic fluids or semen. It is used on all clients indiscriminately and incorporates concepts such as: handwashing before and after each patient contact (See skill 2-4); the use of personal protective equipment or protective barriers such as gloves, gowns, goggles (See skill 2-5) and mouthpieces used in resuscitation efforts; the safe disposal of sharps and needles in approved containers, avoiding recapping of needles; and, the safe disposal of contaminated items and linen (See skill 2-6).

Transmission-based precautions are used with clients who have a known or suspected infection that can be transmitted by airborne, droplet or contact routes. Airborne precautions are used to protect against small-particle droplets that are widely distributed and remain suspended or airborne. These precautions are used when clients are suspected of having tuberculosis, measles, varicella or disseminated varicella zoster virus. These clients require a private room (door closed) with negative air pressure and the use of a filtered mask by caregivers. Droplet precautions, used to protect against larger droplet particles which disperse into air currents, are initiated to prevent the transmission of infections due to Neissaeria meningitides, Haemophilus influenzae, Bordetella pertussis, influenza, and other pathogens that are spread via droplets. These clients need a private room (door may be open) and caregiver must wear a mask when within three feet of the client. Contact Precautions, refer to hand or skin transmissions, and are used for the prevention of infections related to multi-drug-resistant bacteria, and various enteric, viral or parasitic pathogens. These infections can be acquired via direct contact with a client or indirect contact with client care items or environmental surfaces, such as dressings, instruments, dirty gloves or unwashed hands. Hand washing before and after care, as well as use of personal protective equipment (gown, gloves), are required when using contact precautions. This client will be in a private room or paired with a client with the same active infection. Guidelines and common symbols used for transmission-based precautions can be found inside the front and back covers of this book. Additional information may be obtained from the CDC at http://www.cdc.gov/ncidod/hip/ISOLAT/isolat.htm

Hand Washing

Thoroughly washing hands is considered the most important measure to reduce the risk of transmission between individuals. Washing hands immediately before and after contact with clients must be practiced to prevent transmission of microorganisms. The use of gloves does not eliminate the need for hand hygiene. Besides health care workers, visitors should be encouraged to thoroughly wash hands before and after contact with clients. The CDC has developed guidelines for handwashing and alcohol-based handrubs, available at http://www.ede.gov/handhygiene/ and has recommendations that health care facilities develop and implement a system for measuring improvements in adherence to CDC guidelines. Futhermore the CDC has identified risk factors that lead to poor adherence.

Gloves

Following standard precautions, gloves should be worn:

- for touching blood and body fluids requiring standard precautions, mucous membranes, or nonintact skin of all clients, and
- for handling items or surfaces soiled with blood or body fluids to which standard precautions apply.

when any contact with body fluids may potentially be encountered.]

Gloves are changed after contact with each client. Hands and other skin surfaces must be washed immediately, or as soon as client safety permits, if contaminated with blood or body fluids requiring universal precautions. Hands should be washed immediately after gloves are removed. Gloves will reduce the incidence of blood contamination of hands during phlebotomy, but they cannot prevent penetrating injuries caused by needles or other sharp instruments. In addition, the following general guidelines apply:

- Use gloves for performing phlebotomy when the health care worker has cuts, scratches, or other breaks in his/her skin.
- Use gloves in situations where the health care worker judges that contamination with blood may occur (e.g., when performing phlebotomy on an uncooperative client).
- Use gloves for performing finger and/or heel sticks on infants and children.
- Use gloves when persons are receiving training in phlebotomy.

Masks and Gowns

Masks and protective eyewear or face shields should be worn by health care workers to prevent exposure of mucous membranes of the mouth, nose, and eyes during procedures that are likely to generate droplets of blood or body fluids requiring standard precautions. Gowns or aprons should be worn during procedures that are likely to generate splashes of blood or body fluids requiring standard precautions.

Needles and Other Sharp Objects

All health care workers should take precautions to prevent injuries caused by needles, scalpels, and other sharp instruments or devices. Precautions apply during procedures; when cleaning used instruments; during disposal of used needles; and when handling sharp instruments after procedures. To prevent needlestick injuries, needles should not be recapped by hand, purposely bent or broken by hand, removed from disposable syringes, or otherwise manipulated by hand. After they are used, disposable syringes and needles, scalpel blades, and other sharp items should be placed in puncture-resistant containers for disposal. Puncture-resistant containers should be located as close as practical to the use area. All reusable needles should be placed in a puncture-resistant container for transport to the reprocessing area.

Infection Control

General infection control practices should further minimize the already minute risk of a salivary transmission of HIV. These infection control practices include the use of gloves for digital examination of mucous membranes and endotracheal suctioning, hand washing after exposure to saliva, and minimizing the need for emergency mouth-to-mouth resuscitation by making mouthpieces and other ventilation devices available for use in areas where the need for resuscitation is likely. Although standard precautions do not apply to human breast milk, gloves may be worn by health care workers in situations where exposures to breast milk might be frequent (e.g., in breast milk banking).

CONCLUSION

The skills in this book were written with current practice and standards in mind. Nursing practice should not be considered static. Even though minimum standards dictate the basis to practice, ongoing research leads to changes and advancements in practice. With this in mind, it is imperative to note that skill implementation will vary with individual experience and expertise, and will vary between institutions depending on internal outcome measures and research. How a skill is performed may change or be further delineated as new research and knowledge is applied to hands-on care.

Acknowledgments

Dr. Altman would like to acknowledge the tireless efforts and contributions of the staff at Delmar, especially Patricia Gaworecki, Mary Ellen Cox, Robert Plante, Catherine Ciardullo, and Matthew Filimonov.

Further appreciation is extended to the many nurses, contributing authors, and health care personnel who shared their knowledge and experience in writing the skills for this book.

Special recognition is given to the individuals in the photographs, and the clients, families, and health care personnel who so generously allowed staff to photograph them and record their giving and receiving care. During this very personal time photographers were allowed into their milieu.

Special Thanks

The author would like to acknowledge the extensive contributions by the staff at NRSPACE Software who were instrumental in the production of the first edition by providing editing, photography, and overall organization. A special thanks to Valerie Coxon, RN, PhD (CEO), Keith Goodman (Project Manager), Karrin Johnson (Photography and Editorial Assistant), Teri Reed (Photography), and Maja Butler (Editorial Assistant).

Special thanks to Eileen Collins and Hsin-Yi (Jean) Tang for their assistance in investigating current research and changes in practice, revising skills, developing special considerations, critiquing, and editing.

Photography

Photography was provided by NRSPACE Software, Bellevue, Washington and Fabian-Baber Communications, Incorporated who directed and produced the video series of skills to accompany this book.

About the Author

Gaylene Bouska Altman, RN, PhD

Gaylene Bouska Altman is currently the director of the Learning Lab and on the faculty at the University of Washington. Her role includes teaching and coordinating hands-on skills for the nursing courses. She holds a diploma in nursing from Marymount College, Salina, Kansas; a BSN from the University of Kansas, Lawrence; and both an MN and PhD from the University of Washington, Seattle. With more than 25 years of teaching experience, she has taught at both the undergraduate and graduate levels. Besides predominantly teaching at the University of Washington, Dr. Altman has also taught at Seattle University, Seattle Pacific University, and Catholic University (Washington, DC). and has received numerous awards. Most recently Dr. Altman received the 2002 University of Washington School of Excellence in Undergraduate Teaching Award. With a background as an intensive care and coronary care nurse, she has taught courses ranging from fundamental to advanced practice. Her main emphasis has been to develop critical thinking strategies through case presentations. Dr. Altman was one of the pioneers in initiating coronary care units and a mobile coronary care system in the 1970s, in the state of Washington. Furthermore, she helped develop some of the early quality assurance programs implemented throughout the state. Dr. Altman's work has been published in numerous textbooks and journals. She has delivered presentations throughout the country and maintains membership in several professional organizations.

References

Allison, J., Tekawa, I., Ransom, L., & Adrian, A. (1986, January 18). A comparison of fecal occult-blood tests for colorectal-cancer screening. *New England Journal of Medicine, 334*, 155–159.

American Diabetes Association. (1997). Bedside blood glucose monitoring. *Diabetes Care, 20*, (suppl. 1), S53.

Anderson, M. D. (1996). *Fecal occult blood test useful in screening for colorectal cancer. Oncolog, 41*(3). http://audumla.mdacc.tmc.edu/~oncolog/

Association, A. D. (2001, August 25). *Guideline for glucose monitoring.* Available: http://www.cdc.gov/ncidod/hip/Guide/handwash.htm data updated 08-25-01 [2002, May 19].

Association, A. H. (2002). American Heart Association. Available: http://216.185.112.5/presenter.jhtml?identifier=4417 [2002, March 26].

Bayne, G. C. (1997). How sweet it is: Glucose monitoring equipment and interpretation. *Nurse Manager, 28* (9), 52–54.

Cowan, T. (1997). Blood glucose monitoring devices. *Professional Nurse, 12* (8), 593–596.

DeLaune, S. C., & Ladner, P. K. (2002). *Fundamentals of nursing: Standards and practice 2nd edition.* Albany: Delmar.

Greendyke, R. M., & Gifford, R. F. (1996). Bedside blood glucose testing and controlling diabetes mellitus. In letters, *Laboratory Medicine, 27* (9), 565.

Junnila, J., Lassen, P. (1998). Testicular masses. *Am Fam Physician, 57*(4), 685-692.

Kacker, A., Gonzales, D., & Selesnick, S. (1999). The otoscopic examination: What to look for—where to seach. *Consultant, 39*(9), 2397-2398.

Kestel, F. (1996). What's new in blood glucose meters. *Nursing 96, 26* (8), 24.

Lefevre, M. L. (1998). Prostate cancer screen: More harm than good? *Am Fam Physician, 58*(2), 432-438.

Martin, S., Jensen, R., Daly, L., Jergensen, C., Johnson, M. B., & Buell, T. (1997). Comparison of two methods of bedside blood glucose screening in the NICU: Evaluation of accuracy and reliability. *Neonatal Network, 16* (2), 39–43.

Quinn, L. (1998). Glucose monitoring in the acutely ill patient with diabetes mellitus. *Critical Care Nursing Quarterly, 21* (3), 85–96.

Stenger, P., Allen, M. E., & Isius, L. (1996). Accuracy of blood glucose meters in pregnant subjects with diabetes. *Diabetes Care, 19* (3) 268–269.

Voss, E. M., Bina, D. M., McNeil, L. D., Johnson, M. L., & Cembrowski, G. S. (1996). Determining acceptability of blood glucose meters: Evaluating a' blood glucose testing system. *Laboratory Medicine, 27* (10), 679–682.

CHAPTER 1

Physical Assessment

Skill 1-1	Physical Assessment
Skill 1-2	Taking a Temperature
Skill 1-3	Taking a Pulse
Skill 1-4	Counting Respirations
Skill 1-5	Taking Blood Pressure
Skill 1-6	Weighing a Client, Mobile and Immobile
Skill 1-7	Measuring Intake and Output
Skill 1-8	Breast Self-Examination
Skill 1-9	Male Genitalia, Hernia and Rectal Examination
Skill 1-10	Collecting a Clean-Catch, Midstream Urine Specimen
Skill 1-11	Testing Urine for Specific Gravity, Ketones, Glucose, and Occult Blood
Skill 1-12	Performing a Skin Puncture
Skill 1-13	Measuring Blood Glucose Levels
Skill 1-14	Collecting Nose, Throat, and Sputum Specimens
Skill 1-15	Testing for Occult Blood with a Hemoccult Slide

SKILL 1-1

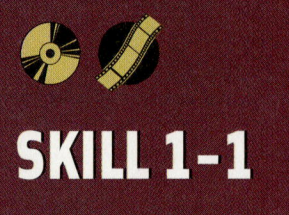

Physical Assessment

Carla A. Bouska Lee, PhD, ARNP C, FAAN,
Claretta D. Munger, ARNP, Valerie Coxon, RN, PhD, and
Eileen Collins, MN, ARNP, CNOR

KEY TERMS

Assessment
Auscultation
Baseline
Examination
Health assessment

Inspection
IPPA
Palpation
Percussion
Physical

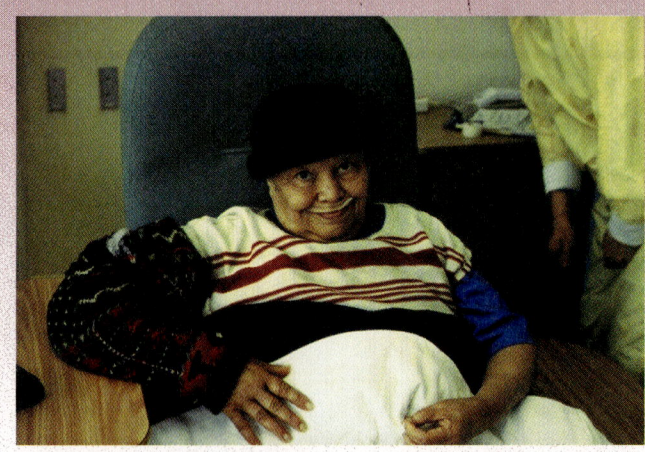

▶ OVERVIEW OF THE SKILL

A dynamic health assessment is the foundation of all nursing care with physical assessment as part of every holistic health evaluation. Assessment is the first step of the nursing process. It involves the orderly collection of objective information about the client's health status. Objective data are observable, measurable, and verifiable by more than one person. A fundamental systematic approach is used based on a combination of head-to-toe and body system assessments. These assessments are expanded as appropriate to the client's situation and setting. By using a systematic approach, one ensures that signs are not overlooked and that time is used efficiently. Through the process of data collection, meaningful information—including health status, actual and potential health problems, and areas of focus for priority health promotion—is identified. Physical assessment/examination is used in outpatient, inpatient, and/or home health services.

A complete and organized assessment is obtained by using a combination of head-to-toe and body system approaches in conjunction with the use of four basic techniques: inspection, palpation, percussion, auscultation (IPPA):

- Inspection: Observation (see, smell); starts during the health history and continues throughout the exam; always comes first (before you touch or listen); continues concurrently with PPA. First, note general observations and then specifics of each area proceeding from the outside to the inside.
- Palpation: Use touch to assess skin temperature, moisture, vibrations and organ or mass location, texture, shape, and size. Identify presence of pain, fluid, or crepitus. First light touch (1 cm), then deep (4-5 cm), rebound (deep with quick release). Compare symmetry for equality, such as the chest (e.g., respiratory vibrations-tactile fremitus).
- Percussion: Done to assess density or aeration. Audible sounds produced by tapping with the hyperextended middle finger on a surface with quick, sharp wrist motion. Tap to produce vibration sounds from light to heavy. Compare areas and symmetry of the body, such as the chest. More solid areas will produce lower pitched sounds, and more air-filled areas will produce higher pitched sounds. Sounds produced:
  - Tympany: loud, high pitch, drum like (example: gastric air bubble)
  - Hyperresonance: very loud, low pitch, booming (example: emphysematous lungs)
  - Resonance: loud, low pitch shallow (example: normal lungs)
  - Dull: medium sound, mid-pitch (example: muscle, bone)
  - Flatness: soft, short duration (example: muscle, bone)

- Auscultation: Listening direct (naked ear) and indirect (acoustical stethoscope or Doppler amplification). Analyzes intensity, pitch, duration, quality, and location. The bell analyzes low-pitched sounds, and the diaphragm analyzes high-pitched sounds.

  A combined body system and body area approach focuses assessment by groupings:
- General Appearance: Examine appearance in the following groups: (1) skin, hair, and nails; (2) head, face, and lymphatic; (3) eye, ear, nose, mouth, and throat; (4) neck and upper extremities; (5) chest, breasts, and axillae; (6) thorax and lungs/respiratory system; (7) heart and cardiovascular system; (8) abdomen/gastrointestinal system; (9) genitalia/genitourinary system and anus.
- Lower Extremities: Musculoskeletal system (MBJB: muscles, bones, joints, and back assessment).
- Neurological: Reflex, sensory, cranial, cerebral, cerebellar, neurodevelopmental, neuropsychiatric.

  Internal genitalia, rectum, and prostate examinations are usually included in advanced assessment and will not be addressed here.

  The IPPA organization can be combined by cephalo-caudal (head-to-toe), general-to-specific, medial-to-lateral, and external-to-internal approaches within each category. The physical assessment is always correlated with the health history as well as with other assessments, such as laboratory or diagnostic data and/or developmental, psychosocial, family, and cultural assessment data. The nurse must also consider her own understanding of anatomy and physiology, basic nursing skills, and the nursing process. The educational preparation and clinical expertise of the nurse may, therefore, influence the extent to which the nurse participates in the physical assessment process.

▶ ASSESSMENT

1. Assess the environment, resources, and the client's medical condition to determine a complete and systematic examination by reducing the possibility of overlooking important findings.
2. Assess the client's history of previous physical assessments and the availability of previous data **to provide a baseline for comparisons.**
3. Assess the client's receptiveness to being examined **to help plan to reduce anxiety and improve compliance with the examination.**
4. Assess the client's understanding of the procedure **to help plan ways to reduce anxiety and improve compliance with the examination.**

▶ DIAGNOSIS

- Disturbed Body Image—if abnormal physical findings.
- Risk for Situational Low Self-Esteem—if abnormal physical findings.
- Deficient Knowledge about normal and abnormal physical findings.

Through the accurate and efficient health assessment process, normal, normal variant, and abnormal data are identified. The nurse can identify serious or life-threatening signs and critical assessment findings that require immediate attention. She/he can utilize the objective data obtained during the physical assessment

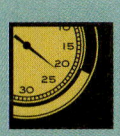

Estimated time to complete the skill: **Variable depending on the purpose and depth of the examination: average of 20–30 minutes.**

process to contribute to problem-solving strategies that identify the client's current health status (acute, chronic, risk, and preventive). The nurse can institute problem-solving strategies to place the client and the client's family or community in optimal health status.

▶ PLANNING

Expected Outcomes:

1. Identify health parameters at multiple levels for total client management and to identify acute concerns and needs.
2. Identify serious, acute, or life-threatening abnormalities or critical assessment findings that require immediate attention.
3. Identify potential or chronic abnormalities that need planned intervention.
4. Monitor chronic stable problems to detect changes from baseline assessments.
5. Identify health risks, concerns, or needs. These include risks that are related to age, gender, environment, community, personal habits, or family history.

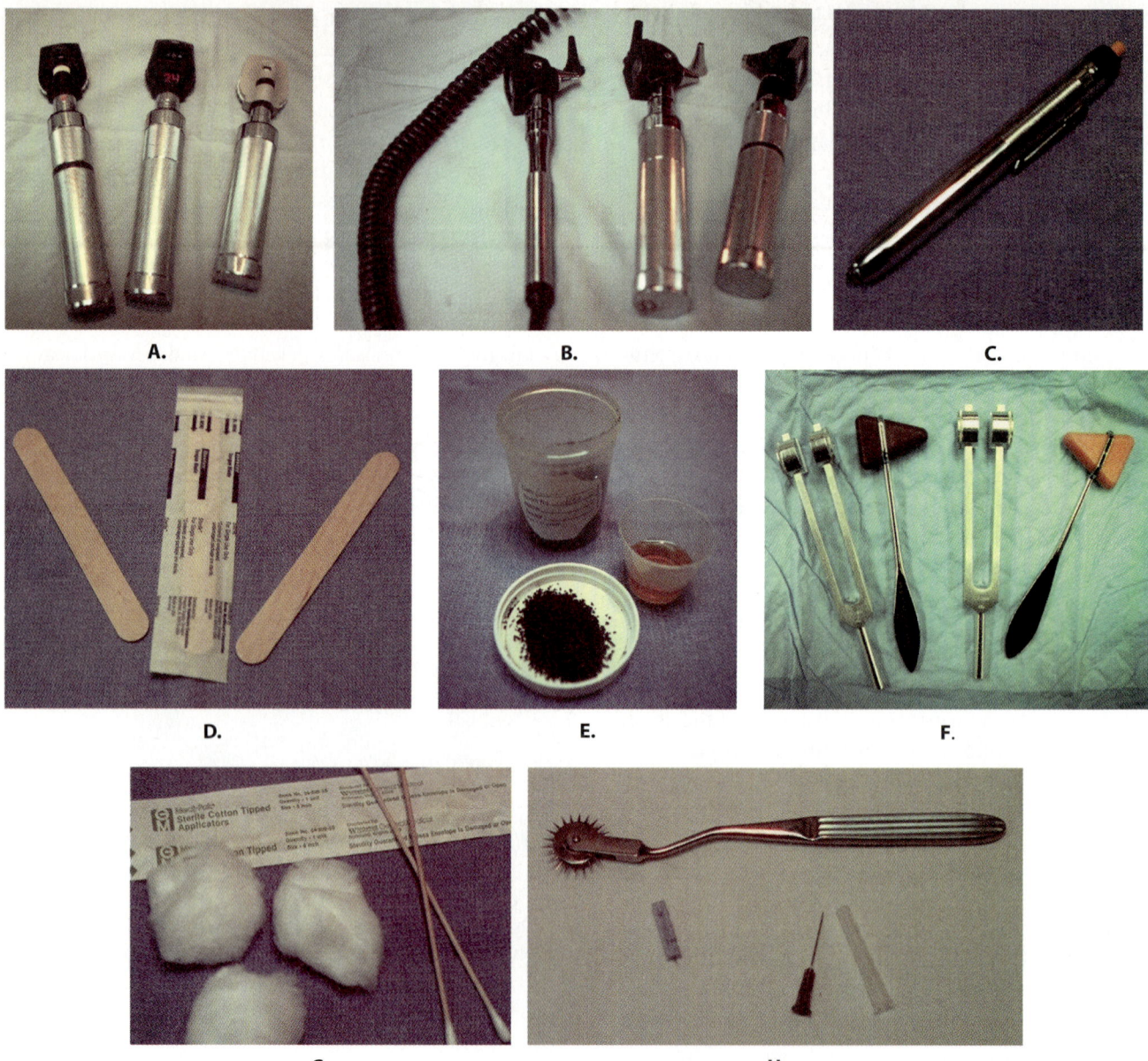

Figure 1-1-1 A. Ophthalmoscopes; **B.** Otoscopes; **C.** Penlight; **D.** Tongue depressors; **E.** Coffee grounds and orange extract; **F.** Tuning forks and reflex hammers; **G.** Cotton swabs and cotton balls; **H.** Sharp items used to assess sharp and dull sensations.

6. Respond to health maintenance needs. This includes monitoring the client's status and comparing findings with normal health parameters for age and gender. It also includes identifying normal variations of health that do not need intervention, providing routine or scheduled assessments, immunizations, preventive or palliative health care, and health education or anticipatory guidance.

Equipment Needed (see Figures 1-1-1A to 1-1-1H):

Equipment must be organized for easy accessibility. It is helpful to be able to reach each piece of equipment with one hand on the client. Short fingernails and warm hands are essential for performing a satisfactory physical examination. Equipment includes the following:

- Pen
- Assessment forms or paper to record notations as well as document findings
- Charts for recording height and weight (and head circumference for infants), age, gender, culture, and sometimes medical condition
- Well-lit, warm, private room or space
- Gown for client privacy and comfort (swimsuits work well with children and adolescents)
- Drape sheet or blanket for client privacy and comfort

- Thermometer: otic or oral/axillary digital preferred
- Stethoscope: acoustical with bell and diaphragm; ideal tubing less than 35 cm long
- Watch with a second hand
- Sphygmomanometer and blood pressure cuff (bladder width to be 40% and length 80–100% of the upper arm circumference)
- Ophthalmoscope
- Vision charts: Illiterate (matching letters or objects), Snellen (far vision), Rosenbaum (near vision) pocket card, Ischara (color vision), or Titmus tester (includes all four), and pupil gauge (in mm)
- Otoscope with pneumatic tube
- Audio testing equipment: watch, tuning forks (minimum of one high pitched, 512 Hz, and one low pitched, 128 Hz), handheld audiometer, tympanometer, or full audiometry with soundproof room
- Nasal speculum with illumination. Optional headlamp with magnification
- Penlight
- Tongue depressors
- Nonsterile gloves (possibly sterile gloves as well)
- Glass of water
- Marking pen
- Measuring tape (with cm and inches), preferably cloth or plastic
- Water-soluble lubricant
- Guaiac card for occult blood
- Specimen cup
- Reflex hammer
- Neurological "kit": temperature (test tubes of hot and cold), touch (cotton ball, hair pin, paper clip, safety pin, key, marble, coin, low-pitched tuning fork), taste (sweet—sugar, honey; sour—lemon, lime, vinegar; bitter—alum, quinine; salty—salt, saline), smell (coffee, lemon, orange extract, flowers, perfume, mouthwash). If making your own kit, be sure to use identical appearing containers for each category and a cotton-tipped applicator or dropper for consistent application.
- Other (these are helpful to have available although are not always used): slide, toothbrush (helpful to obtain skin scrapings), Wood's lamp, magnifying glass, small test tube, flashlight and transilluminator, head lamp, gooseneck lamp, Doppler (for amplification of body sounds), goniometer, Denver Developmental Screening Kit contents, Mini-mental status exam, fluid-resistant gowns, masks and eye covers.

▶ CLIENT EDUCATION NEEDED

1. Introduce yourself by name and title. In some cases you may need to describe your role as well.
2. Provide the client with an explanation of what is to follow (I will be checking everything from your head to your toes) and an approximate time frame for the exam. It helps to tell children how they will know when you are done (e.g., when I tell you to put your shoes back on).
3. Inform the client if you will be jotting down notations during the examination and how these will be used. This reassures confidentiality.
4. Before performing each step in the physical assessment process, inform the client of what to expect, where to expect it, and how you anticipate it will feel (I don't think any of this will hurt but be sure to tell me if it does hurt).
5. Inform the client of what you are looking for and why as you perform your physical assessment. You can accomplish a great deal of education about the body, how it functions, and health prevention while performing your examination.
6. Teach skin self-examination as you evaluate the skin.
7. Teach breast self-examination as you examine breasts (male and female).
8. Teach testicular self-examination and self-checking for hernias during the genital exam.
9. Teach proper urinary hygiene and basics about sexually transmitted diseases (STDs) with the genital exam.
10. Reinforce good hygiene as you wash your hands and conduct the examination.

▶ DELEGATION TIPS

Physical assessment skills are within the practice realm and licensure of the Registered Professional. The nurse is responsible for instructing ancillary personnel to report any changes in the client's physical appearance or condition to the nurse for further assessment and evaluation. The nurse is responsible to instruct ancillary personnel to report any changes in the client's physical appearance or condition to the nurse for their assessment.

IMPLEMENTATION—ACTION/RATIONALE

ACTION	RATIONALE
1. Organize equipment.	1. Promotes efficiency.
2. Review the client's medical history (see Figure 1-1-2).	2. The first step of holistic assessment. Provides important clues on which to focus or follow up during physical assessment.
3. Wash hands, preferably in front of the client.	3. Reduces transmission of microorganisms. Educates the client.
4. Explain the plan and procedure.	4. Educates the client. Reassures the client.
5. Assist the client to a sitting position, if possible.	5. Provides best access to begin examination.
6. Examine the client.	6. Collects information about health and disease.
7. Present any appropriate findings. Ask for additional information. Answer the client's questions.	7. Provides closure for the examination and communicates information.
8. Schedule follow-up assessments, tests, or other appointments as needed.	8. Provides for follow-up care.
9. Clean, replace, and discard equipment appropriately.	9. Promotes efficiency, organization, and reduces microorganisms.
10. Wash hands.	10. Reduces the transmission of microorganisms.

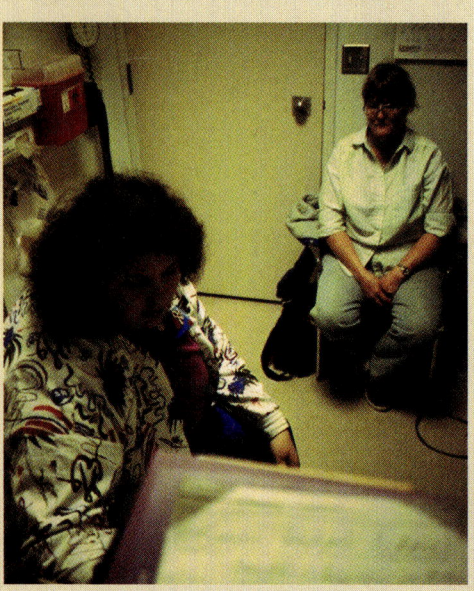

Figure 1-1-2 Review client history. Clients are often uncomfortable and anxious in the unfamiliar clinic setting. Establishing privacy and using words and body language to create a supportive environment help place the client at ease. Listen to the client's complaint, ask pertinent questions about symptoms and medical history, and write down key information.

Measurements and Overall Observations

11. Obtain baseline measurements and compare with normal data. Remember that normal values vary with age and normal temperatures do not rule out illness, especially with very young and elderly clients.
    Check height, weight, head circumference (check normal values based on age percentiles for infants to 24 months), and temperature (palpate skin temperature during examination as well).

12. Measure the heart rate, rhythm, and volume; the respiratory rate and rhythm; and the blood pressure bilaterally.

13. Check anthropometric measurements prn, body mass index (BMI), etc.

14. Assess the overall appearance of the client in a "once over" evaluation before you begin the detailed examination. Look for clues to poor health, such as level of consciousness, personal hygiene, nutritional status, posture, gait, symmetry, appearance, and appropriateness of clothing. Listen to the quality and appropriateness of speech. Observe facial expressions, if the client makes eye contact, and how comfortable the client is with interpersonal interaction.
    Assess whether age is congruent with appearance. Observe body fat, stature, motor movements, and body and breath odors.
    Assess dress, grooming, personal hygiene, speech, facial expressions, general mannerisms, mood and affect.
    Look for signs of distress, as evidenced by breathing patterns, speech, facial expressions, perspiration, tension, guarding, bracing, and anxiety.

11. Provides measurable objective data about health state or baseline data.

12. Provides clues for additional observations or actions required later in the examination.

13. Body mass and height-weight proportion can be better indicators of illness than simple height and weight measurements.

14. Provides objective clues about overall health state and clues to possible specific abnormalities to watch for later in the examination.

Skin, Hair, and Nails Examination

15. Take a moment to assess initially and continue assessment as you perform the remainder of the exam.
    - Inspect: color, vascularity, lesions, ulcers, scars, hair distribution, nail shape and configuration, nail bed angles. Measure, describe, draw, and/or stage abnormalities.

15. Detects normal variation and abnormalities. Establishes a baseline for future comparisons. Skin abnormalities, including crepitus, nodules, mobility, and hydration will provide clues to illness, and are often indicators of systemic abnormalities.

continues

Skin, Hair, and Nails Examination *continued*

- Palpate: moisture, temperature, texture, turgor, capillary refill (normal capillary refill is less than 3 seconds), edema.

Head, Face, and Lymphatics Examination

16. Inspect and palpate the head, face, and lymph nodes (see Figures 1-1-3 and 1-1-4). Proceed front to back.

17. Head: Examine scalp, hair, and cranium (frontal-parietal-temporal-occipital). Examine fontanelles and sutures in newborns to 24 months. Head should be normocephalic and symmetrical with no acromegaly, hydrocephalus, craniosynostosis, premature closure of sutures, masses, depressions, tenderness, or infestations.

18. Lymph nodes: Examine preauricular, postauricular, occipital, submental, submandibular, anterior cervical chain, posterior cervical chain, tonsillar, supraclavicular, and parotid. Lymph nodes should be less than and nontender. Note that children may have multiple nodes less than especially postauricular, but these will be small, nontender, and movable.

19. Temporomandibular joint: Observe the motion of opening and closing the jaw. It should articulate smoothly without crepitus, clicking, or tenderness. There should be no sign of inflammation.

20. Face: Observe for shape, symmetry, and expression. Have the client smile, frown, raise eyebrows, wrinkle forehead, show teeth, purse lips, puff cheeks, press tongue into cheek, "cluck" tongue and whistle. Inspect, percuss, and palpate frontal and maxillary sinuses. Use a wisp of cotton to assess tactile sensation over the trigeminal nerve sites and mandible bilaterally.

    Facial features should be symmetrical with a nasolabial fold present bilaterally. Clients of Asian descent may have slanted eyes with inner epicanthal folds. Normal sounds should be resonant. No pain should be present on percussion or palpation.

    Abnormal findings include edema, disproportionate structures, or involuntary movements.

---

16. Confirms health and identifies signs and symptoms of illness or disease, infections, old or new trauma, or other abnormalities.

17. Confirms health and identifies signs and symptoms of illness or disease, infections, old or new trauma, or other abnormalities.

18. Confirms health and identifies signs and symptoms of illness or disease, infections, old or new trauma, or other abnormalities.

19. Confirms health and identifies signs and symptoms of illness or disease, infections, old or new trauma, or other abnormalities.

20. Confirms health and identifies signs and symptoms of illness or disease, infections, old or new trauma, or other abnormalities.

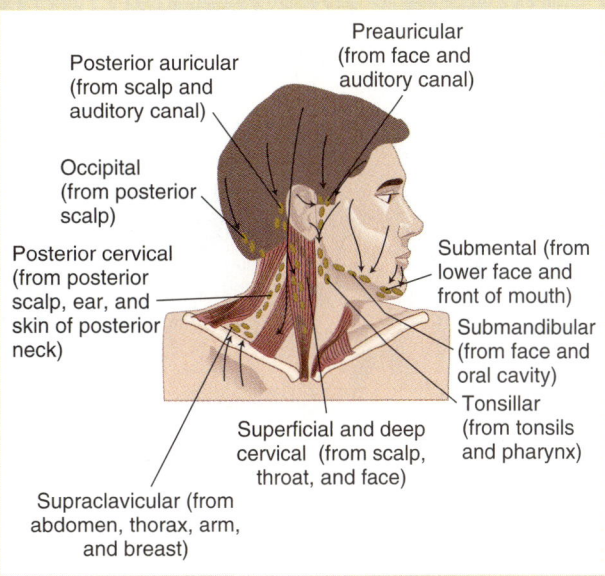

Figure 1-1-3 Lymph nodes of the head and neck. Arrows indicate drainage patterns.

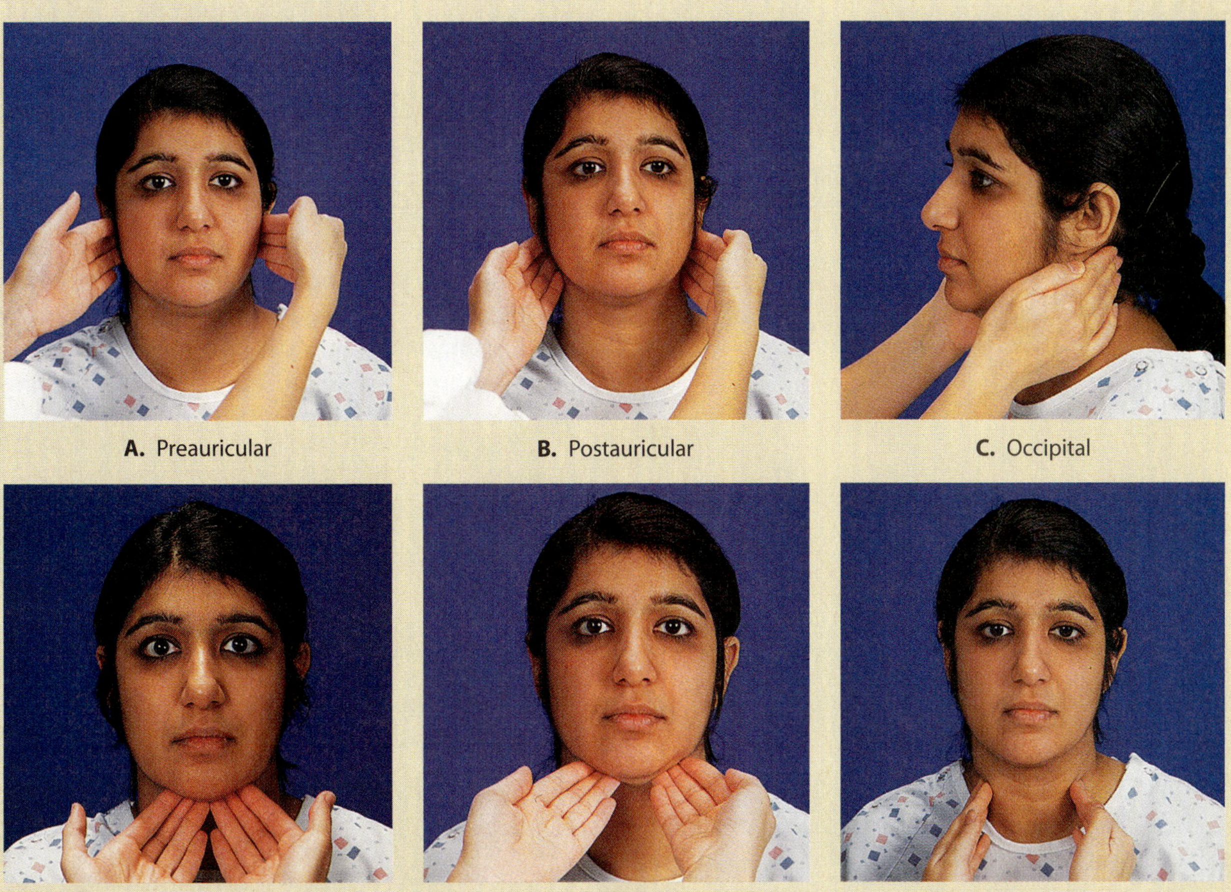

| A. Preauricular | B. Postauricular | C. Occipital |
| D. Submental | E. Submandibular | F. Anterior cervical chain |

Figure 1-1-4 Palpation of lymph nodes *(continues)*.

continues

Head, Face, and Lymphatics Examination
continued

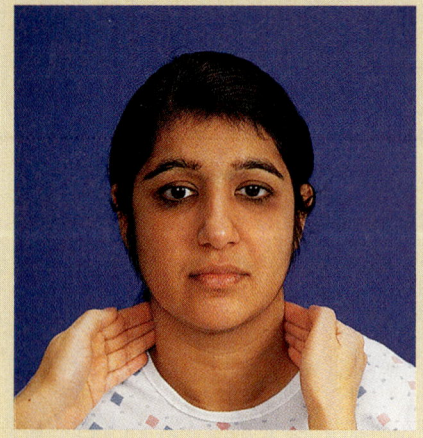 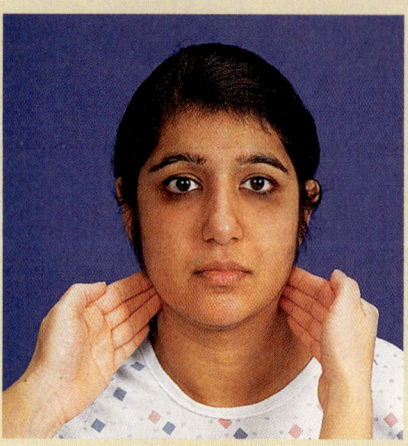 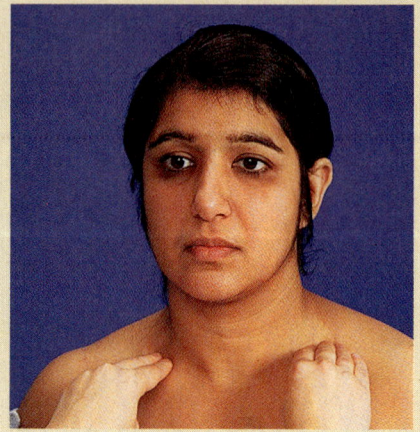

  G. Posterior cervical chain   H. Tonsillar   I. Supraclavicular

Figure 1-1-4 Palpation of lymph nodes.

Eye, Ear, Nose, Mouth, and Throat Examination

21. Examine the eyes. Inspect and palpate external structures, including brows, lids, lacrimal gland, and puncta. Inspect eye position and palpebral fissures. Examine bulbar and palpebral conjunctivae, sclera, cornea, and iris. Assess for a corneal touch reflex.

21. Confirms health and identifies signs and symptoms of illness or disease.
- Establishes the presence or absence of drooping, infection, or tumors. Confirms that the lid "meets" the iris, the lid margins are smooth, tears flow evenly instead of accumulating and "tearing up" the eye.
- Establishes the presence or absence of inflammation of hair follicles, hemorrhages, discharge, discolorations, ectropion, swelling, edema, blepharitis, or dacryoadenitis.
- Checks that the third cranial nerve (CN III) raises the lids symmetrically, and that the puncta are open and without inflammation.

22. Extraocular mobility: Check for Hirschberg's corneal light reflex using the cover-uncover test. Check the six cardinal fields of gaze. Examine pupils, including size, shape, response to light and accommodation, both direct and consensual. Examine the lens and retinal structures. First check for a red reflex with the ophthalmoscope set on "0." Move the diopter wheel to "+" to focus on anterior ocular structures and "−" to focus on posterior structures. Locate the retina, vessels, optic disk, and macula.

22. Checks that light reflects symmetrically from the center of corneas at 12–15 inches, and that the uncovered eye stays focused.
- Checks the functions of CN III, IV, and VI.
- Checks for the absence of tropia, phoria, or nystagmus.

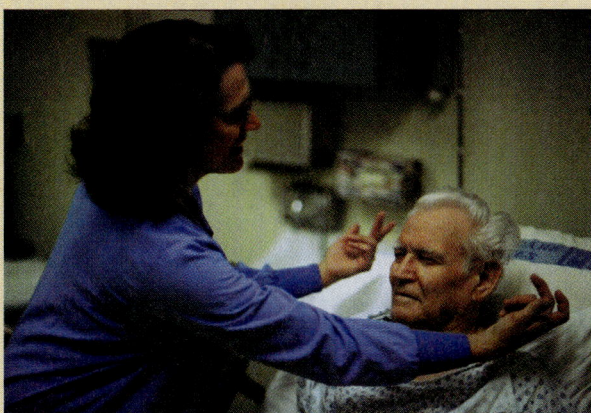

Figure 1-1-5 Have client identify the moment an object enters the visual field.

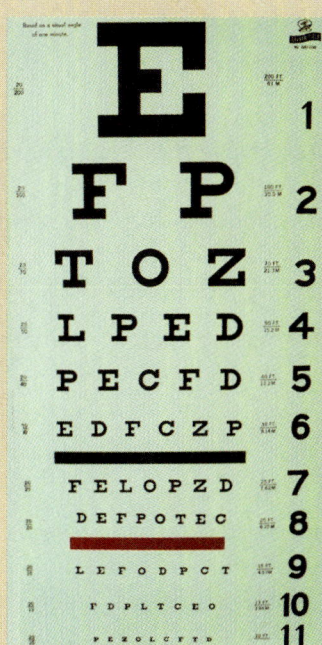

Figure 1-1-6 Snellen chart used to assess visual acuity.

23. Have the client identify an object, such as your finger, as it enters the visual fields from each of four directions. Normal movement is temporal 90 degrees, nasal 60 degrees, superior 50 degrees, and inferior 70 degrees (see Figure 1-1-5).

24. Check for visual acuity, including near and far sight, primary colors, and Ishihara plates (see Figure 1-1-6).

25. Examine the ears. Inspect and palpate the external ear, including alignment, pinna, tragus, lobule, and neck mastoid muscle. Observe the shape, color, and size of the ear.

26. Proceed with an otoscopic assessment, starting with the ear canal. Identify landmarks, the tympanic membrane, and observe tympanic membrane movement. Use tympanometry if needed to confirm visual findings.

27. Check the client's hearing acuity. Note responses to normal sounds. In an infant, observe for a startle reflex/bell response. In adults, conduct a voice/whisper or watch-tick test at 1–2 feet. Conduct Weber and Rhinne tests at 512 Hz.

23. Checks the function of CN II.

24. Visual acuity tests are the last step in the eye examination so that physical abnormalities that might cause abnormal acuity will be detected first.

25. Confirms health and identifies signs and symptoms of illness or diseases of the ear. Checks for normal alignment, that the top of the ear crosses an imaginary line from eye to occiput. Checks for abnormal findings of tags, excess wax, drainage, deformities, nodules, inflammation, pain, and a tender or "boggy" mastoid.

26. Establishes the quality of tympanic membrane (TM) movement, detects retractions, bulging, and abnormal or discolored middle ear fluid. Confirms if there are signs of infection, impaction, or other abnormalities.

27. Hearing acuity tests are the last step in the ear examination so that physical abnormalities that might cause abnormal acuity will be detected first.

continues

Eye, Ear, Nose, Mouth, and Throat Examination *continued*

28. Examine the nose. Inspect and palpate for nasal patency. Have the client inhale and exhale through each nostril. Observe the external surface, nasal mucosa, turbinates, and septum.

28. Confirms health and identifies signs and symptoms of illness or disease, including unusual or excessive discharge, damaged septum, polyps, tenderness, or nonclear drainage.

29. Have the client identify common odors.

29. Tests CN I (the olfactory nerve).

30. Examine the mouth, including the teeth, tongue, and throat (see Figure 1-1-7).

30. Confirms health and identifies signs and symptoms of illness or disease.

31. Inspect and count teeth.

31. Confirms the number and condition of teeth for age.

32. Inspect and palpate lips and frenula, gums, buccal mucosa, tongue protrusion and frenulum, salivary glands, hard and soft palates, tonsils, uvula position and movement, and arches. Inspect the naso-oro-pharynx.

32. Identifies lesions, color of membranes, abnormalities, cavities, odors, swelling, inflammation, swallowing difficulties, or hyperplasia.

33. Conduct gag reflex response, and taste tests for sweet, sour, bitter, and salt.

33. Tests cranial nerve functions.

34. Examine the neck. Inspect and palpate the trachea. Check that the trachea runs midline down the neck by examining the trachea at the suprasternal notch.

34. Confirms health and identifies signs and symptoms of illness or disease.

35. To examine the thyroid, observe the anterior neck slightly extended, then have the client flex the neck and swallow. Palpate the anterior neck, then palpate forward from the posterior. Identify tracheal rings, isthmus, thyroid cartilage, and gland lobes as the client is swallowing.

35. Checks for goiter, nodules, enlargement, or tenderness in the neck and thyroid.

36. Palpate the temporal and carotid pulses. Assess the quality, character, rhythm, and strength of the pulse.

36. Identifies signs and symptoms of cardiovascular illness or disease.

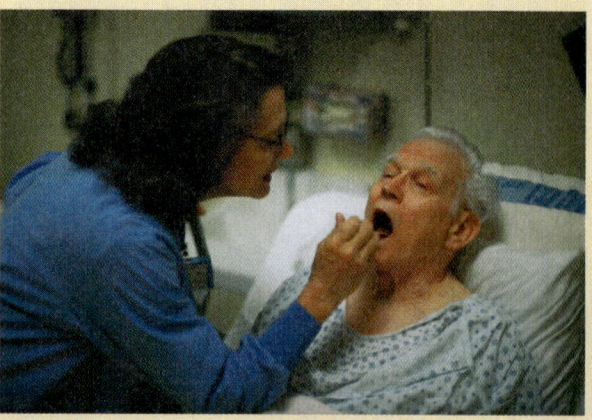

Figure 1-1-7 The mouth examination includes the teeth, tongue, throat, oral mucosa, and salivary glands.

Upper Neuromuscular Examination

37. Inspect and palpate muscles, bones, and joints. In general, evaluate from the periphery to the center of the body.
    Observe the configuration, symmetry, size, tone, and range of motion (ROM). Assess strength using resistive ROM.

38. Examine the cervical spine. Flex, extend, move lateral, and rotate the spine. Examine the spine for resistive strength by pushing your hand against the side of the client's face. Push left, right, back on the forehead, forward on the occiput, and down on the top of the head.

39. Examine shoulders. Flex, hyperextend, abduct, adduct, turn in internal and external rotation, shrug, and push/pull against the shoulders.

40. Examine elbows. Flex, extend, rotate, push, and pull each elbow.

41. Examine wrists. Flex, extend, and rotate each wrist.

42. Examine hands by having the client grasp your hands with his/hers.

43. Examine fingers. Abduct and adduct the fingers. Perform finger thumb opposition with counting and position sense.

44. Examine the epitrochlear lymph nodes, brachial and radial pulses, and bicep, tricep, and brachioradialis reflexes.

Chest and Breast Examination
(See Skill 1-8, Breast Self-Examination)

45. Inspect and palpate the breast, nipple, and areola. Palpate the axillary lymph nodes.

46. Calculate the Tanner stage of sexual maturity if appropriate.

47. Repeat breast and axillae examination while the client is in the supine position.

---

37. Confirms health and identifies signs and symptoms of illness or disease.

38. Checks the cervical spine, sternocleidomastoid, and trapezial baseline strength, integrity, and function.

39. Detects limitations of mobility, torticollis, pain, crepitus, nodules, lumps, or pulsations in the muscles, bones, and joints.

40. Checks for tenderness and mobility.

41. Checks for tenderness and mobility. Detects the presence of carpal tunnel.

42. Checks for tenderness and mobility.

43. Checks for tenderness and mobility.

44. Confirms that lymph nodes are nonpalpable and nontender, and that pulses are strong and regular. Checks neurological reflexes.

45. Confirms health and identifies signs and symptoms of illness or disease. Detects lumps, nodules, or discharge in tissue. Detects tenderness or lumps in axillary nodes, which drain the chest and breast.

46. The Tanner stage assesses appropriate breast development progression and status for age and provides an opportunity for teaching.

47. Repeating the examination while the client is supine increases likelihood of early identification of abnormalities.

continues

Back and Posterior Lung Examination

48. Inspect and palpate the skin.

48. Confirms health and identifies signs and symptoms of illness or disease.

49. Recheck the thyroid from the posterior position.

49. Gland lobules are easier to palpate from back.

50. Examine the cervical and thoracic spine (see Figure 1-1-8), the scapulae, and the rib cage. Observe the posterior thoracic expansion. Estimate the anteroposterior-to-transverse chest ratio. A normal ratio is 1:2.

50. Determines normal, normal variations, and abnormal findings in alignment, flexion, spinous processes, and paravertebral muscles. Checks that the scapulae are equal, and the rib cage is symmetrical.

51. Feel for the presence of fremitus posteriorly and laterally. Compare sides.

51. Checks for fremitus either increased with consolidation, or decreased with hyperinflation of the lungs. Bilateral comparison enables identification of differences.

52. Use indirect percussion at a minimum of four sites, preferably in regular intervals every 5 cm from top to bottom of lung fields. Move from superior to inferior and from lateral to spine.

52. Indirect percussion allows comparison of resonance bilaterally, and checks for tenderness over the lungs and kidneys. The organized sequence of side to side and superior to inferior increases the possibility of detecting abnormalities.

53. Auscultate the lungs (see Figure 1-1-9) using a side-to-side sequence and moving down 2–5 cm at a time. Listen to inspiration and expiration at each site. Listen for vocal fremitus while the client makes "99" and sustained "ee" sounds.

53. Checks for bronchial noises over trachea, bronchovesicular sounds in the first and second intercostal spaces (ICSs), and vesicular sounds over the peripheral chest. Detects abnormal sounds of rales, rhonchi, or wheezes.

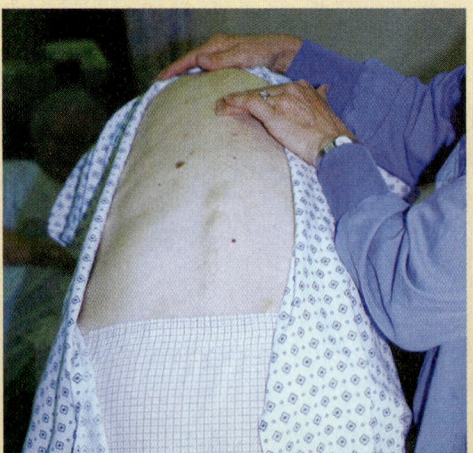

Figure 1-1-8 Examine the cervical and thoracic spine for alignment, flexion, and symmetry with the rib cage and scapulae.

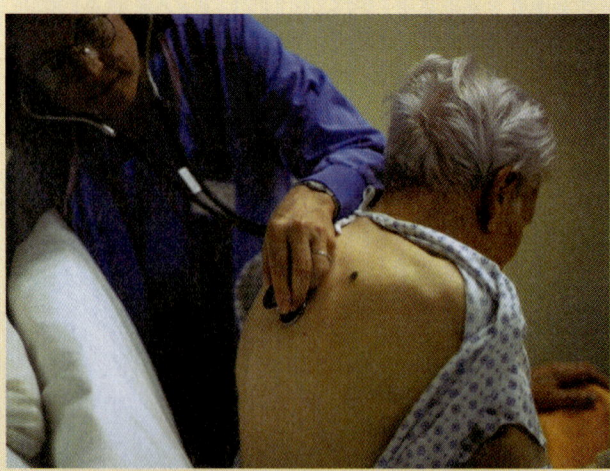

Figure 1-1-9 Auscultate the lungs, listening to inspiration and expiration at each site.

Thorax, Lungs, and Respiratory Examination

54. Stand in front of the client.

55. Inspect and palpate the anterior chest. Observe position, chest movement, size, shape, and symmetry of the clavicles and ribs.

56. Listen to the respiratory rate, including rhythm and depth of respirations. Compare rate with normal respiratory rates for the age of the client.

57. Observe the diaphragmatic excursion, ICSs, respiratory muscles, respiratory effort, and expansion. Watch for pursed lips, cyanosis, or a cough. Note that abdominal breathing is normal from birth to 2 years of age.

58. Feel for tactile fremitus along the lung apexes and bases.

59. Use indirect percussion at intervals over ICSs, moving superior to inferior and collateral to spine. Percuss lung apexes and bases, and the cardiac border if appropriate. Note that percussion should be resonant over the lung, flat over bone, and dull over organs.

54. Prepares to examine anterior lungs.

55. Confirms health and identifies signs and symptoms of illness or disease. Checks for barrel chest, pectus excavatum, pectus carinatum, or tripod "splinting" positions. Splinting positions indicate the client is compensating for decreased oxygenation.

56. Checks for 2:1 timing of the exhale/inhale breathing cycle. Detects shortness of breath (SOB), and abnormal respiration patterns, including Cheyne-Stokes, tachypnea, hyperpnea, and hyspnea (see Figure 1-1-10).

57. Detects accessory muscle use or stridor.

58. Detects fremitus, which is increased with consolidation or decreased with hyperinflation.

59. Side-to-side and superior-to-inferior organized approach increases the possibility of detecting abnormalities.

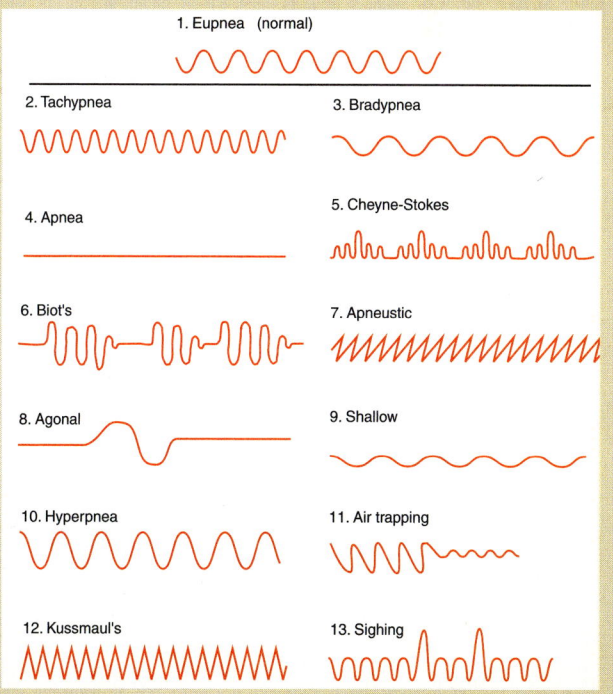

Figure 1-1-10 Normal and abnormal respiratory patterns.

continues

Thorax, Lungs, and Respiratory Examination *continued*

60. Auscultate the anterior lung fields, using the same progression as the palpation procedure. Avoid listening over bone and breast tissue. Observe intensity, pitch, ratio, quality (see Figure 1-1-11).

Listen for vocal fremitus during "99" and sustained "ee" sounds (egophony or whispered pectoriloquy).

60. Checks for bronchial noises over trachea, bronchovesicular sounds to the left and right of the sternum in the first and second ICSs, and vesicular sounds over the peripheral chest. Detects abnormal sounds of rales, rhonchi, or wheezes.

Heart and Cardiovascular System Examination

61. Inspect and palpate the precordium. Identify the point of maximal intensity (PMI) at the mitral/apical area of the heart. This pulsation, associated with ventricular contraction, is located at the left fifth ICS. Confirm synchrony with the carotid pulse. The PMI may be visible in children and thin clients. Palpation of the PMI in large or muscular persons may require leaning the client forward or to the left side.

61. Confirms health and identifies signs and symptoms of illness or disease. Confirms the absence of cardiomegaly symptoms, visible thrills, heaves, and pulsations (except possibly 1–2 cm movements at mitral area during systole, especially in children, thin clients or elderly clients).

62. Auscultate with the client sitting, then leaning forward. Listen with the diaphragm and then the bell.

62. The bell detects lower pitched sounds than the diaphragm.

63. Auscultate the apical heart rate and feel radial pulse at the same time. Identify rate, rhythm, regularity, amplitude, and difference between apical and radial pulses. Note carotid impulse with apical sound.

63. A difference in apical and radial pulse (pulse deficit) reflects difference in stroke volume with each beat. Irregular rates with pulse deficit may indicate atrial fibrillation, whereby disorganization exists between atrial and ventricle electrical activity.

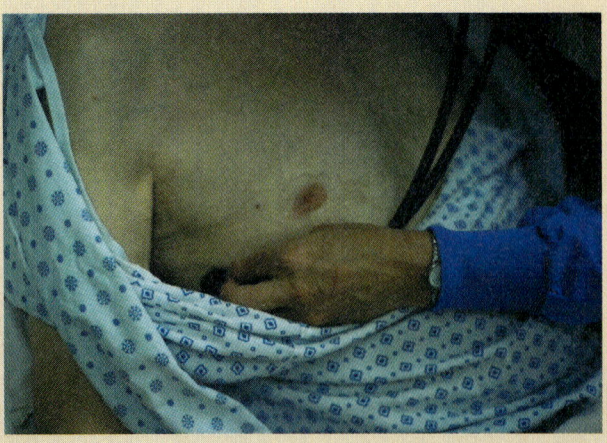

Figure 1-1-11 Auscultate the anterior lung fields. Listen for abnormal sounds, including rales, rhonchi, or wheezes.

64. Examine all valvular landmarks at least twice. First locate and identify the S1, S2, S3, and S4 heart sounds. Then listen for other sounds (murmurs, rubs, clicks, etc.). Auscultate in an orderly fashion from the apex to the base of the heart (or vice versa).	64. Systematic progression of the examination minimizes omissions. Detects normal physiology, as the S_1 closure of mitral and tricuspid valves heralds the onset of systole. Detects any abnormal opening snap in early diastole, which could indicate mitral stenosis.
65. In the mitral area identify that S_1 is louder than S_2 with the diaphragm of the stethoscope, because the left heart pressure is greater than the right, and the mitral valve closes slightly before the tricuspid valve. Use the bell to listen for a possible S_3 sound (see Figure 1-1-12).	65. Detects S_3 sounds, which are early diastolic filling sounds from the ventricles, and could indicate diastolic gallop.
66. In the tricuspid area, identify that S_1 is louder than S_2 with diaphragm, but that it is softer than at the mitral area. Listen for possible S_1 split that disappears when the client holds his/her breath. Listen for the S_3 sound with the bell.	66. Detects the normal aortic valve closure occurring slightly before the pulmonic valve closure during inspiration as more negative intrathoracic pressure causes an increase in venous return to the right side of the heart.
67. In the pulmonic area identify that S_2 is louder than S_1, but softer than at aortic area. Note that physiologic splitting of S_2, which indicates closure of the semilunar valves at this site is normal. In the aortic area identify that S_2 is louder than S_1 with diaphragm.	67. Finds symptoms of abnormal splits, which are wide, fixed, or paradoxical.
68. Assess the epigastric, axillary, and Erb's point areas.	68. Assesses for signs of mitral valve prolapse, which are best heard at the epigastric location. Assesses for abnormal murmurs radiating to the axilla. Checks Erb's point where both aortic and pulmonic murmurs may be heard.
69. Summarize the character of S_1 and S_2 sounds. Note the presence or absence of S_3 and S_4 (gallop), murmurs, rubs, clicks, or snaps.	69. S_3 can be normal in children, in the third trimester of pregnancy, and adults younger than 30 years old. Other sounds need investigation.
70. Assist client to left lateral position to continue the cardiac examination.	70. Positions the heart closer to the chest wall.
71. Auscultate mitral and tricuspid sites with the bell.	71. Mitral and tricuspid abnormalities are heard best in the left lateral position.
72. Assist client to return to supine position and continue cardiac examination.	72. Facilitates next portion of cardiac examination.

continues

Heart and Cardiovascular System Examination *continued*

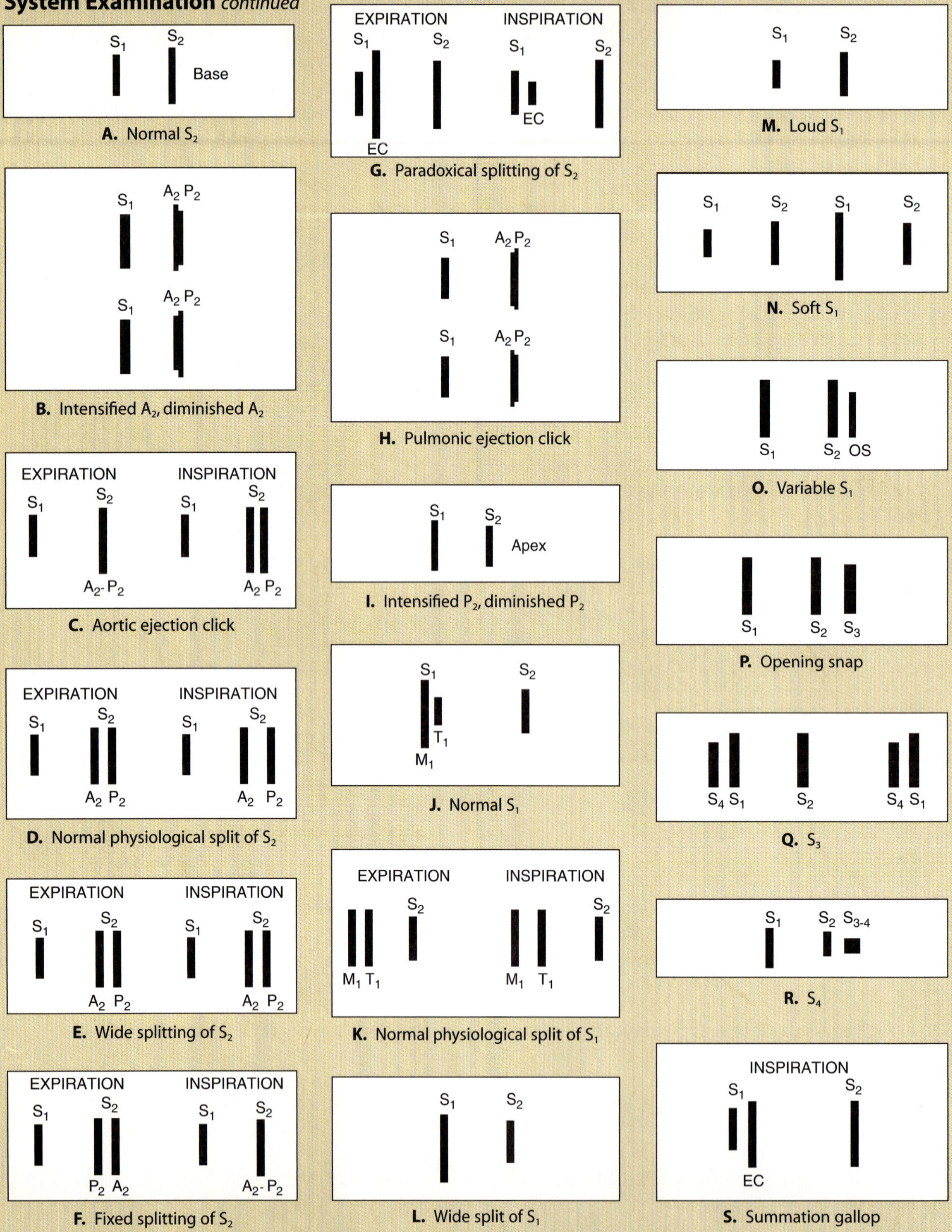

A. Normal S_2

B. Intensified A_2, diminished A_2

C. Aortic ejection click

D. Normal physiological split of S_2

E. Wide splitting of S_2

F. Fixed splitting of S_2

G. Paradoxical splitting of S_2

H. Pulmonic ejection click

I. Intensified P_2, diminished P_2

J. Normal S_1

K. Normal physiological split of S_1

L. Wide split of S_1

M. Loud S_1

N. Soft S_1

O. Variable S_1

P. Opening snap

Q. S_3

R. S_4

S. Summation gallop

Figure 1-1-12 Normal and abnormal heart sounds.

73. Inspect and palpate the precordium. Identify the PMI at the mitral area and confirm synchrony with carotid pulse. Assess apical, carotid, temporal, brachial, radial, femoral, popliteal, posterior tibial, and dorsalis pedis pulses (see Figure 1-1-13).
    Percuss the cardiac borders, if needed. Auscultate the heart in supine position with bell, then with diaphragm. Check the mitral, tricuspid, pulmonic, aortic, and ectopic areas. Auscultate with bell for bruits at carotid and temporal pulse sites.

74. Raise head to an angle of 30–45 degrees, and inspect the jugular vein distention (JVD).

Abdominal Examination

75. Inspect the size, contour, and symmetry of the abdomen. The normal abdomen is flat (except in young children), symmetrical, without scars, striae, masses, nodules, peristalsis (except in very thin clients), or rectus ridge (except in young or thin clients). Note pigmentation, scars, striae, masses, nodules, the condition of the umbilicus, and any respiratory or peristaltic movement. Check the rectus abdominus muscle by having the client raise his/her head.

73. The PMI is best palpated in the supine position. Confirms the absence of visible thrills, heaves, and pulsations except possibly a small (1–2 cm) area at the mitral location during systole, especially in children, thin clients, and elderly clients. PMI may not be palpable in large and muscular clients.
    The client's position determines which sounds are heard best. It is easier to hear some murmurs with the client in the supine position. The bell is best for detecting deeper sounds.
    Notes unusual symmetry, rate, rhythm, pulsations, volume, or thrills of pulses.
    Evaluates for cardiomegaly.

74. Detects normal jugular vein distention, which is usually 1–2 cm above the sternal angle when the head is elevated 45 degrees and is usually absent at 90 degrees and distended when flat. Jugular vein pressure (JVP) measurement plus 5 cm will give an estimate of the central venous pressure (CVP).

75. Confirms health and identifies signs and symptoms of illness or disease.
    Aortic pulsations may be seen in epigastric area in thin clients. Newborn to 2 year olds breathe with their abdominal muscles, with no retractions of the intercostal muscles during inspiration, and a smooth rhythm. The unbilicus is normally depressed.

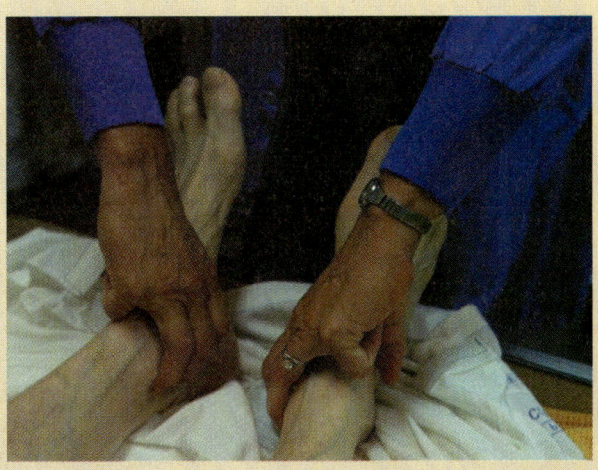

Figure 1-1-13 Assess for unusual symmetry, pulsations, volume, or thrills of pulses.

continues

Abdominal Examination *continued*

76. Auscultate with the diaphragm and then the bell. Listen for bowel sounds in each of the four quadrants. Right lower quadrant (RLQ), right upper quadrant (RUQ), left upper quadrant (LUQ), and left lower quadrant (LLQ).

77. Percuss the RLQ, RUQ, gastric bubble, spleen, bladder, LLQ, LUQ, and liver span (see Figure 1-1-14).
    Note the spleen, located between the sixth and tenth rib, may go undetected. The gastric air bubble (LUQ) is lower pitched than tympany of the intestine. The tympany changes to dull at lower edge of liver, and lung resonance changes to dull at upper edge of liver. You may try to percuss the kidney posteriorly while the client is sitting, if needed.

78. Palpate all four quadrants superficially first then deep and rebound palpations to identify any discomfort, tenderness, or abnormalities. Check superficial abdominal reflexes in the LLQ, LUQ, spleen (use bimanual palpation), RLQ, RUQ, liver, aorta, kidney (use bimanual technique), and bladder (see Figure 1-1-14). Evaluate for guarding on expiration.

79. Check femoral pulses and superficial and deep inguinal nodes.

External Genitalia Examination

80. Assist client to modified or full lithotomy position.

76. Auscultate before palpating, as sounds will change in response to touch.
    Detects a normal frequency of sounds of 5–30 sounds per minute, or abnormal bruits, hums, or rubs.

77. Detects size and location of internal organs as tympany changes to dull over organs.

78. Checks for normal umbilical deviation toward the direction of palpation stroke.
    Determines normal abdomen, which is smooth and soft with no masses, bulges, swelling, organomegaly, bladder distention, fluid retention, or pain. Locates normal findings of palpated liver edge, aortic pulsations, and lower pole of kidney.
    Normal voluntary muscle guarding ceases on expiration.

79. Determines normal pulses, which are symmetrical and even, with no bounding or thrills, and normal inguinal nodes, which are less than 1 cm, movable, and nontender.

80. Lithotomy position without stirrups is usually more comfortable for the client; however, both positions provide good visibility and access.

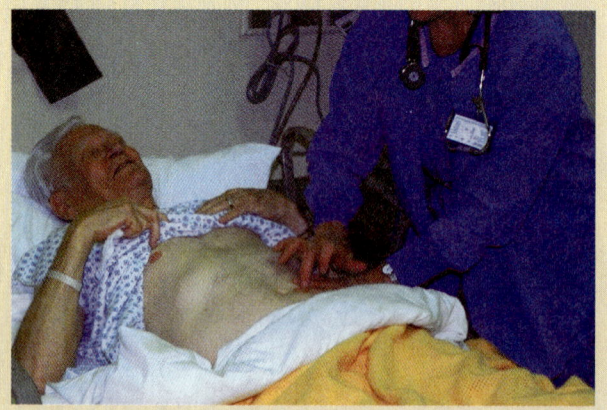

Figure 1-1-14 Percuss the abdomen to assess size and location of internal organs.

81. Inspect and palpate deep inguinal nodes.

82. Observe pubic hair distribution, color, and texture. Check the femoral and inguinal areas for hernias.

83. Calculate the Tanner stage of sexual maturity if appropriate.

84. Check the skin and look for abnormalities. In women, examine the mons pubis, labia majora, labia minora, clitoris, urethral meatus, vaginal introitus, and perineum.

85. In men, check the cremasteric reflex (in infant), urethral meatus, penis (glans, foreskin, shaft), scrotum (transilluminate if hydrocele suspected), scrotal rugae, testicles, epididymis, spermatic cord, and external inguinal ring.

86. Examine the anus. You may need to return the client to the left lateral position or have the client stand and lean elbows on the exam table to aide in visualization.

Lower Extremity and Musculoskeletal Examination

87. Assist the client down from the table to a standing position, if necessary.

88. Have the client walk across the room while observing his/her gait. Observe from the side profile, assessing cervical, thoracic, and lumbar curves. Look for differences in height of shoulders, iliac crests, and skin creases below the buttocks. Ask the client to bend forward as you observe the spine for any curvatures or deformities. Check the range of motion (ROM) of the spine. Have the client bend forward to touch toes (flexion), bend sideways (lateral bending), and then bend backward (extension). Stand beside the client for support if needed. Check

81. Deep nodes are more easily palpated in this position.

82. Confirms normal distribution of hair in an inverse triangle, and identifies abnormalities, including infestations, rashes, edema, condylomata, vesicles, varicose veins, discharge, odor, or bulges.

83. The Tanner stage assesses appropriate genital development progression and status for age and provides an opportunity for teaching.

84. Checks for abnormal color, lesions, pain, trauma, abnormal size, imperforate introitus, odor, or discharge.

85. Confirms normal appearance, where the urethral meatus is located centrally, with dorsal vein prominence, a small amount of smegma, and the left scrotal sac lower than the right. Detects a nonretractable foreskin in an uncircumcised child.
    Checks for abnormal lesions, odor, swelling, inflammation, nodules, condyloma, vesicles, pustules, scaling, edema, phimosis, chordee (curvature), hernia, hydrocele, spermatocele, or varicocele.

86. Confirms normal appearance of sacral dimpling, dark pink to brown color, puckered, and free of lesions, swelling, inflammation, tenderness, itching, fissures, rashes, masses, hemorrhoids, or skin tags.

87. Observe the client's ability to change position and assist for safety when needed.

88. Observe if gait is steady and assess if the client is at risk for falls. The normal spine has concavities in the cervical and lumbar regions and a convexity in the thorax. If iliac crests are uneven, it is suggestive of unequal leg lengths. Scoliosis may be noted if there is deviation in the line from T1 to the gluteal cleft. Decreased spinal mobility may be noted in osteoarthritis as well as other conditions.
    When a paravertebral muscle is in spasm it looks prominent, feels tight, and is tender to the touch.

continues

Lower Extremity and Musculoskeletal Examination *continued*

rotation as the client twists from side to side.
   Palpate the paravertebral muscles for tenderness and spasm.

89. Assist the client to the supine position.

89. Prepares for the next sequence in the examination.

90. Inspect and palpate the skin. Look at the skin color, check that capillary refill is less than 3 seconds, observe hair distribution, veins, temperature, and texture of skin.
   Observe the size, shape, isometric muscle contraction, tone, and strength (using resistive ROM) of muscles.

90. Detects skin atrophy, breakdown, edema, ulcerations, or varicose veins.
   Determines that muscle shape is symmetrical, with good tone. Detects atrophy, hypertrophy, flaccidity, spasticity, spasm, masses, or involuntary movements.

91. Inspect the joints. Palpate from periphery to center. Observe contour, periarticular tissue, neutral anatomic position, ROM (active and palpate passive), and strength (resistive motion). Also evaluate the hips. Have the client do a straight leg raise. Move the hips knee to chest, internal rotation, external rotation, abduction, and adduction. Listen carefully for a hip click in infants (Ortolani's sign).
   Assess the knees. Check the tibiofemoral joints by flexing the knee 90 degrees and with thumbs palpate tibial margins and collateral ligament. Check knee flexion, extension, and strength.
   For the ankles and feet, palpate the Achilles' tendon, at-rest, in dorsiflexion and plantar flexion, eversion and inversion. Check toe flexion, abduction, and adduction. Palpate metatarsophalangeal joints and interphalangeal joints.
   Check popliteal, posterior tibial, and dorsalis pedis pulses.

91. Confirms joints articulate in proper alignment and are free from swelling, nodules, pain, warmth, deformities, masses, crepitus, grating, or popping.
   Evaluates for contractures, pain, or swelling.

   Evaluates for clonus, varus, valgus, planus, deviations, and inflammation.

Neurological Examination

92. Assist the client to a sitting position.

92. Prepares for the remainder of the neurological examination.

93. Check for deep tendon reflexes, biceps, triceps, brachioradialis (if not done previously), patellar, and Achilles' reflexes.
   Check infantile reflexes, including rooting, suck, palmer grasp, tonic neck, stepping, plantar grasp, moro, Gallant and Landau.

93. Measures the degree and speed of response, from 0 (absent) to 4+ (hyperactive), and the presence of clonus.
   Observe fanning of toes with stroke of outer aspect of sole of foot from heel across ball.

Check the Babinski reflex. A positive Babinski reflex is normal until walking or 18 months of age.

94. Examine the client's sensory abilities. Check for responses to skin sensations. Begin distally and move proximally. Touch fingers, hands, lower arms and toes, feet, legs, and abdomen as necessary. Be careful not to be "predictable." Alter the rate and rhythm of stimulation.

    Compare right to left and proximal to distal sensations.

    Check exteroceptive sensation, including light touch (use a cotton wisp), and sharp and dull (use a hair pin or paper clip). If the sharp/dull evaluation was abnormal, check temperature sensation as well.

    Check the propioceptive sensations of vibration, motion, and position.

    Check the cortical sensations of stereognosis (coin, button, key, paper clip, etc.; different object in each hand), and graphesthesia. If needed, examine two-point discrimination and extinction. Normal distances vary with the body part tested. For example, fingers are approximately 5 mm, the hand or foot is 20 mm.

95. Review and recheck the cranial nerves:
    CN I: Olfactory

    CN II: Optic

    CN III: Oculomotor

    CN IV: Trochlear

    CN V: Trigeminal motor and sensory

    CN VI: Abducens

    CN VII: Facial motor and sensory

    CN VIII: Acoustic cochlear and vestibular

    CN IX: Glossopharyngeal motor/sensory
    CN X: Vagus motor and sensory

94. Confirms health and identifies signs and symptoms of illness or disease. Confirms normal sensory perceptions.

    Proximal nerve transmission must be functional for distal sensations to be present.

    Determines that client can feel stimuli, detect vibrations over bony prominences (this decreases after age 65), and identify changes in body position and motion. Clients should be able to identify objects with eyes closed.

95. Identify normal versus abnormal functions:
    CN I: To verify the client is able to distinguish and identify odors with each nostril.
    CN II: To verify the client has normal visual acuity, visual fields, and a normal fundus or optic disk.
    CN III: Checks for normal pupil reactions, cardinal fields of gaze, and eyelid elevation.
    CN IV: Checks for normal extraocular movement.
    CN V: Checks for strength and function of temporalis and masseter muscles, trigeminal nerve sensation, including light pain, light touch, temperature, and corneal reflex.
    CN VI: Checks for normal extraocular movements, cardinal fields of gaze.
    CN VII: Checks facial movements (frown, raise eyebrows) symmetrical (no palsy), and tearing.
    CN VIII: Checks for normal hearing, Weber and Rinne tests. Checks vertigo, nystagmus, and good equilibrium.
    CN IX and CN X: Checks for uvula rise midline, speech clear, swallow, taste in posterior third of tongue. Gag present.

continues

Neurological Examination continued

CN XI: Spinal accessory

CN XII: Hypoglossal
A helpful acronym for the cranial nerves is:
On **O**ld **O**lympic **T**owering **T**ops **A** **F**in **A**nd **G**erman **V**iewed **S**ome **H**ops.

CN XI: Checks for shoulders, trapezius, and sternocleidomastoid muscle movements.
CN XII: Checks for clarity of speech and tongue movements.

96. Evaluate the client's mental status. Check level of consciousness, orientation to person, time, place, general appearance, behavior, affect, speech, content, memory, logic, and abstract reasoning (describe proverb), judgment, spatial perception (copy figures, identify familiar sounds, identify right versus left body parts). Mentally summarize the mental status from earlier observations during the examination.

96. Identifies normal versus abnormal functions. Check that the client is awake, alert, and oriented to time and place, and exhibits appropriate behavior. Look for abnormal findings of drowsiness, lethargic, stuporous, comatose, or disoriented behaviors.

97. Examine cerebellar status: Conduct a finger-to-nose test (have the client use the index finger to touch your finger, held 18 inches away from the client, then have client touch his nose). Have client repeat this movement, gradually increasing the speed.
   Observe for the client's ability to cross the midline. Look for tremor, overshoot, and undershoot. Repeat with the other hand.
   Conduct a rapid alternating hand movements (RAHM) and note if the client exhibits smooth pronation-supination with increasingly rapid speed. Have the client touch fingers-to-thumb, and note if he/she can touch thumb to each of the fingers of the same hand in rapid succession from index to fifth finger and back. Note that ability depends on age.
   Have the client touch heel-to-shin, foot taping rapid alternating hand movements (RAHM), and foot "figure 8" movement tests. Determine whether the client can run heel down the shin of the opposite leg.
   Look for smooth rapid ankle extensions and rotation.

97. Confirms health and identifies signs and symptoms of illness or disease. Confirms cerebellar status by evaluating coordination, balance, and checking for smooth and harmonious movement.

98. Assist the client to a standing position.

98. Prepares the client for remainder of examination.

99. Inspect and/or palpate posture, weight-bearing and standing spine alignment, spinous processes, paravertebral muscles, and ROM (flexion, lateral bending, rotation, hyperextension). Do a Romberg test. Balance on the one

99. Determines that shoulders and hips are level, scapulae and iliac crests are symmetrical, toes and knees point forward, extremities are proportionate. Confirms that head spinous processes and gluteal cleft are in

foot for 10 seconds. Repeat heel-to-shin test, and have client hop on each foot and do shallow knee bends.

100. Assess mobility by having the client perform a casual gait, toe and heel walk, tandem walk (forward and backward), step right, step left, walk briskly, and do jumping jacks (if client's condition permits).

101. Recheck heart and respiratory sounds after exercising.

102. Compare the client's status to age-appropriate standards for activities of daily living (ADLs), gross and fine motor function, speech and language, and personal-social interaction.

103. Evaluate for psychiatric symptoms, including disturbed affect, aversive eye contact, symptoms of depression or anxiety, disrupted or confused thought processes, indications of delusional thoughts, and indications of suicidal thoughts.

alignment. Checks for scoliosis, kyphosis, lordosis, or contractures.

100. Assesses cerebellar and developmental status as well as musculoskeletal structure and function.
   Checks that the posture and gait are erect, balanced, smooth, tandem for age with usually less than 1–2 inches between heel to toe steps. Estimates exercise tolerance for age and diagnosis.

101. Checks for flow murmurs, cardiac rate, and recovery time. Compare with resting rates.

102. Confirms health and identifies signs and symptoms of illness or disease.

103. Checks that verbal and nonverbal behavior is consistent and congruent, that there is no evidence of delusions, hallucinations, or suicidal ideations.

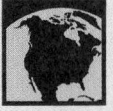

▶ **REAL WORLD ANECDOTES**

A nurse was doing a routine physical assessment on a client with chronic pulmonary disease, listening to lung sounds. She heard a rapid, irregular heartbeat as well. She reported her findings to the nurse-practitioner, who ordered follow-up diagnostic tests. The client was later diagnosed with multifocal atrial tachycardia.

▶ **EVALUATION**

- Client relates history in logical, sequential manner. Questions are answered appropriately and without distraction. Client is able to easily and accurately recall history and facts.
- Explain findings to client within nurse's scope of practice and function.
- Formulate problem list reflecting findings.
- Generate intervention plan.

▶ **DOCUMENTATION**

Client's Chart
- All assessments and procedures must be completely documented according to institutional policy.
- Record under objective portion of assessment.
- Record in order of the category groupings used in the assessment.
- Record date and time of assessment.
- Identify information and historian.

- Indicate ability of client to assist with assessment.
- Record chief concern.
- List positive findings first followed by significant negative findings for each body system or body part examined.
- Record detailed description of assessment related to chief concern (need for visit).
- Record detailed description of abnormalities (positive findings).
- Record description of negative findings.

▶ CRITICAL THINKING SKILL

Introduction

The client knows his own body. Often the client is the expert consultant.

Possible Scenario

A nurse was doing a routine physical exam. While the nurse was concentrating on the priorities in the exam, the client mentioned that he could feel a lump in his hamstring. He wondered if he had injured it jogging. Because the nurse was examining the client's lungs, he listened to the client's complaint, made a noncommittal comment, and continued with his assessment. The client did not bring up his concerns again.

Possible Outcome

One month later, this client was diagnosed with a rhabdomyosarcoma, a highly malignant soft tissue cancer most often seen in children. He underwent surgery, chemotherapy, and radiation, and continues to be evaluated for recurrence every 3 months.

Prevention

This man's survival was directly related to the stage of the disease at diagnosis. This cancer is often found when the client or a parent mentions feeling a lump. The nurse missed the abnormal finding, because he did not follow up on the client's comment. The nurse should have followed up on the complaint by asking for more specifics and history, examining the area carefully, and reporting the findings.

▶ VARIATIONS

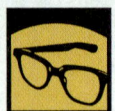

Geriatric Variations:
- *Vital signs and measurements must be age correlated to establish what "normal" is for an elderly client.*
- *Allow extra time for slower movement in an older client.*
- *An elderly client may need a warmer room to feel comfortable.*
- *You will find more "normal variations" in the geriatric population. This is especially true for skin conditions.*
- *Activities of daily living history needs to be assessed in view of visual, auditory, musculoskeletal, and neurological findings.*
- *Any client with a change in neurological function must be evaluated for dementia, depression, Alzheimer's disease, and Parkinson's disease.*
- *Make sure elderly clients can hear and understand what you want them to do when performing the neurological part of the examination.*

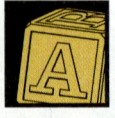

Pediatric Variations:
- *Keep parents within view of the child.*
- *Infants and young children may be more comfortable being examined in a parent's lap. Sit facing the parent with your knees touching theirs to make a "table."*
- *Examine ear, nose, and throat last because the child may react to the invasiveness of the procedures.*
- *Allow the child some play time with your stethoscope or penlight. Clean these items before and after.*
- *Show the child the equipment before using it. Shine the otoscope light in the child's hand.*
- *Blow the air from the pneumatic tube. Sometimes demonstrating the procedure using a toy or doll helps make the child more comfortable.*

▶ VARIATIONS continued

- *Give the child simple choices when possible. Do not bribe. Be honest.*
- *Allow children to cry or yell. Do not allow them to kick or bite.*
- *If there are two children to be examined, let them sit side by side and examine each body area on one and then on the other. You can enlist their cooperation by letting one child watch or help with the other child. Keep a careful recording of abnormal findings so you do not mix up who had what finding.*
- *Remember to thank the child for helping, cooperating, or just for coming in.*
- *Ask teens "private" questions by whispering or lowering your voice without drawing undue attention to the topic and without conveying the idea that certain topics should not be discussed with parents. You can act as a role model or help the child discuss "embarrassing" topics with the parents.*
- *Unclothe a child as you proceed with an examination rather than all at once. Shirt off, examine top half. Shirt on and pants off for bottom half. Leave underpants on, if possible.*
- *Examine the genitalia through a leg hole or by pulling the pants down halfway rather than taking off pants all the way. If you need to remove the underpants, let the child stand up on the table and hug a parent for balance while you perform the exam.*
- *Empower the child after the genital exam by asking the child to perform kicking motions of "exercise" while you check hips and knees. Sit the child up as soon as possible. Sit down to check reflexes, so that you are physically lower than the child, if possible.*

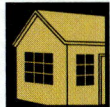

Home Care Variations:
- *The examination can be done in bed, on a couch, or a kitchen table, or even on the floor. Ask the client for suggestions and decide the best location based on the age and flexibility of the client.*
- *Good lighting is more important that an optimum "table" or bed. Consider bringing extra lighting, such as a gooseneck lamp.*

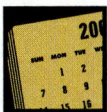

Long-Term Care Variations:
- *Examinations in the long-term-care setting are usually performed with the client in bed. Be sure of good lighting and take your own equipment, if needed.*
- *Auditory and visual privacy is usually more of a problem in this setting. Anticipate schedules and be sure the staff and roommates know how much private time you need.*

▶ COMMON ERRORS

Possible Error:
Skipping seemingly insignificant areas and thereby missing significant information.

Prevention:
Allow enough time for the examination. Ask the client to communicate concerns. Have a systematic progression that covers all areas.

Possible Error:
Failing to follow the sequencing of techniques or omitting one of the techniques such as inspection or palpation.

Prevention:
Bring a checklist into the examination and follow it. Before moving on to the next part of the exam, review in your mind if you have covered all the techniques required to assess the current area.

▶ NURSING TIPS

- Vocalize "a" (like apple) versus "ah" (aw) to get higher uvula rise and better pharyngeal visualization.
- Measure chest circumference, divide by one-half, and subtract transverse diameter for anteroposterior (AP) measurement.
- If you detect rhonchi on auscultation, ask client to cough, then listen again. With infants and older children check lung sounds after performing the gag reflex portion of the pharyngeal exam.
- The heart exam can be a good opportunity to teach the client about the heart. Ask the client to tell you about the heart, where it is located, its size, and its shape. Answer questions about "what a heart attack is" and teach about heart-healthy diet and exercise.
- Follow a specific order when conducting the heart examination: mitral, tricuspid, pulmonic, aortic, ectopic (epigastric and axillary), or vice versa. Remember the order with the mnemonic phrase "**Mom Tries Pasta Again Every Evening.**" You may remember the four heart valves (in reverse order) using the phrase "**A Poor Tired Monkey.**"
- Exercise may make flow murmurs easier to hear.
- Percuss up to lower edge of liver and down to upper edge. Start palpation 2 cm below lower percussed margin and "rock" up and under the rib to look for the edge.

▶ SPECIAL CONSIDERATIONS

- *Observe the client's affect. Provide an open attitude to facilitate receiving information that the client may want to share. A victim of domestic violence may wish to seek help so the examiner should be mindful of potential verbal and nonverbal cues. Clients who abuse alcohol or drugs usually will not readily admit this information; therefore, questions regarding alcohol and drug use can be incorporated into nutrition and medication history. Ask open-ended questions since a quick denial of alcohol or drug use may arrest further questioning. Clients may have health concerns that they wish to discuss. Always ask the reason for contacting a health care provider (routine checkup, s/s of concern) and if there are any further concerns before leaving the room.*
- *Note the client's stress level and realize that it may be a signal for further exam, i.e., cardiovascular.*
- *Breast exams may be performed in a variety of ways. You may see a "roll" method where the hand never leaves the breast. The finger pads roll back and forth across the breast from sternum to axilla and advance about an inch with each forward motion. Some practitioners believe this to be a more accurate approach because no area is missed, as when hands are raised to reposition in other methods. Most lumps are found behind the nipple and in the upper outer quadrant. Special attention should be paid to these areas during the exam.*

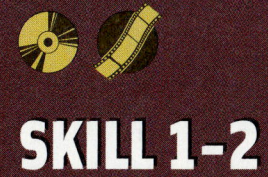

SKILL 1-2

Taking a Temperature

Karrin Johnson, RN and Gaylene Bouska Altman, RN, PhD

KEY TERMS

Antipyretic
Axillary
Centigrade
Fahrenheit
Hypothermia
Oral
Pyrexia
Rectal
Thermometer
Tympanic

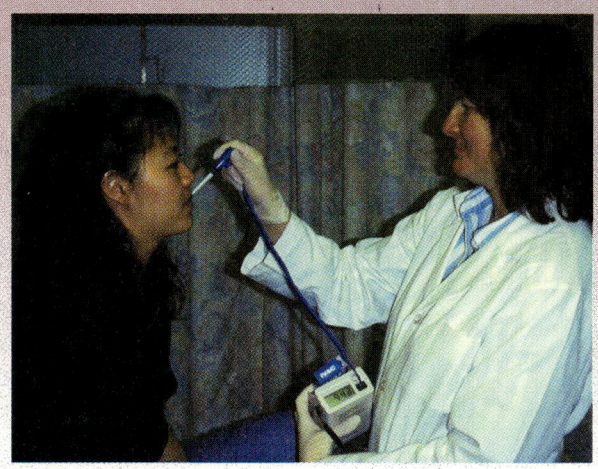

▶ OVERVIEW OF THE SKILL

Monitoring body temperature is a basic skill necessary in nursing and medical decision making. When heat production exceeds heat loss, and body temperature rises above the normal range, pyrexia (fever) occurs. Pyrexia can accompany any inflammatory response, loss of body fluid, or prolonged exposure to high temperatures. When the body is exposed to temperatures lower than normal for a prolonged length of time, hypothermia occurs. Hospitalized clients are at particular risk for infection and accompanying fever. Clients are stressed by their presenting conditions, and their bodies are further stressed by the hospital environment; thus, they are more susceptible to the infectious agents found there. Hypothermia generally occurs in response to prolonged exposure to cold weather or as a result of being immersed in cold water. Accurate monitoring and recording of a client's temperature is essential for diagnosis, treatment and monitoring of the client.

▶ ASSESSMENT

1. Assess body temperature for changes when exposed to pyrogens (endogenous or exogenous substances that cause fever) or to extreme hot or cold external environments **because such environments may indicate the cause of an infection**.
2. Assess the client for the most appropriate site to check temperature **in order to obtain an accurate reading**.
3. Confirm that the client has not consumed hot or cold food or beverage nor smoked for 15 to 30 minutes before the measurement **because these activities may alter the oral reading**.
4. Assess for mouth breathing and tachypnea **because both can cause an inaccurate oral reading**.
5. Assess for oral lesion, especially herpetic lesions **because herpes viruses are extremely contagious and require implementation of Standard Precautions of the Centers for Disease Control and Prevention. Clients with herpetic lesions should have their own glass thermometer or disposable thermometer to prevent transmission to others**.

▶ DIAGNOSIS

- Ineffective Health Maintenance. The patient may have increased risk of exposure to pyrogens (surgery, medical procedure, injury, or illness).
- Risk for Infection. The patient may have signs or symptoms of infection.

CHAPTER 1 Physical Assessment

- Hypothermia.
- Hyperthermia.
- Ineffective Thermoregulation.
- Deficient Fluid Volume.

▶ PLANNING

Expected Outcomes:

1. An accurate temperature reading will be obtained.
2. The client will verbalize understanding of the reason for the procedure.

Equipment Needed (see Figure 1-2-1):

- Thermometer (one of the following)
  — Electronic thermometer with disposable protective sheath
  — Tympanic membrane thermometer with probe cover
  — Disposable, single-use chemical strip thermometer
  — Glass (mercury free): oral or rectal at client's bedside usually color coded to avoid cross use.
- Lubricant for rectal and glass thermometer

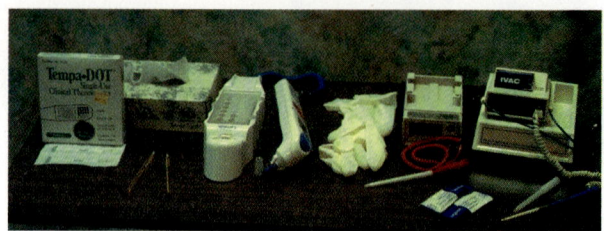

Figure 1-2-1 Many types and brands of thermometers are available to assess temperature.

- Two pairs of nonsterile gloves
- Tissues

▶ CLIENT EDUCATION NEEDED

1. Explain to client why an accurate body temperature is needed.
2. Describe the equipment to the client and explain what to expect during the procedure.
3. Answer any questions and/or fears the client may have regarding the procedure.

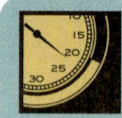 Estimated time to complete the skill: **5–10 minutes.**

▶ DELEGATION TIPS

The skill of temperature measurement is often delegated to ancillary personnel; however, the nurse retains responsibility for knowledge of the client's temperature and appropriate actions. The expectation is that ancillary personnel will have documented instruction and competency validation of their ability to:

- *Select the correct route for measurement of the temperature*
- *Correctly position the client for measurement*
- *Correctly perform the measurement according to established guidelines and record on the appropriate flow sheet (clinical record)*
- *Recognize and report abnormal findings appropriately*

IMPLEMENTATION—ACTION/RATIONALE

ACTION	RATIONALE
1. Review medical record for baseline data and factors that influence vital signs.	1. Establishes parameters for client's normal measurements, provides direction in device selection, and helps determine site to use for measurement. Vital signs are measured in the order of temperature, pulse, and respiration (TPR) and

SKILL 1-2 Taking a Temperature

2. Explain to the client that vital signs will be assessed. Encourage the client to remain still and refrain from drinking, eating, and smoking. Avoid mouth breathing, if possible.

3. Assess client's toileting needs and proceed as appropriate.

4. Gather equipment.

5. Provide for privacy.

6. Wash hands and apply gloves when appropriate.

blood pressure (BP), usually without interruptions, to provide the nurse with an objective clinical database to direct decision making.

2. Encourages participation, allays anxiety, and ensures accurate measurements. Cold or hot liquids and smoking alter circulation and body temperature. Mouth breathing can alter temperature.

3. Prevents interruptions during measurements, communicates caring, and promotes client comfort.

4. Facilitates organized assessment and measurement.

5. Decreases embarrassment.

6. Hands are washed before and after every contact with a client to reduce the transmission of microorganisms. Gloves are worn to avoid contact with bodily secretions and to reduce transmission of microorganisms.

Oral Temperature—Electronic Thermometer

7. Repeat Actions 1–6.

8. Place disposable protective sheath over probe (see Figure 1-2-2).

7. See Rationales 1–6.

8. Reduces transmission of microorganisms.

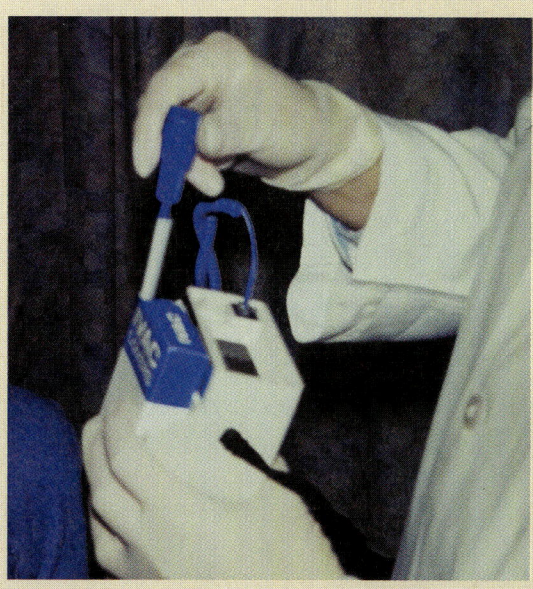

Figure 1-2-2 Place disposable sheath over probe.

continues

Oral Temperature— Electronic Thermometer *continued*

9. Grasp top of the probe's stem. Avoid placing pressure on the ejection button.

10. Place tip of thermometer under the client's tongue and along the gumline to the posterior sublingual pocket lateral to center of lower jaw (see Figure 1-2-3).

9. Pressure on the ejection button releases the sheath from the probe.

10. Sublingual pocket contains superficial blood vessels.

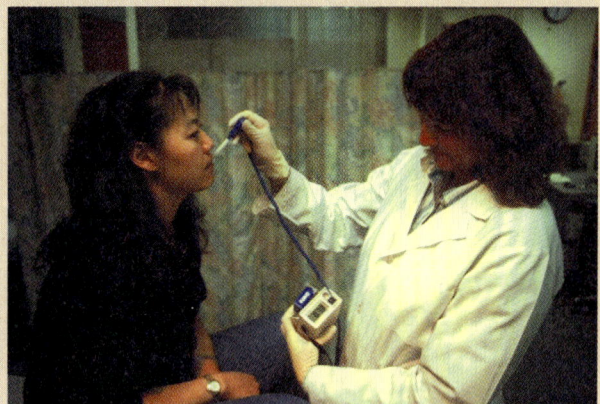

Figure 1-2-3 Place probe tip in the posterior sublingual pocket.

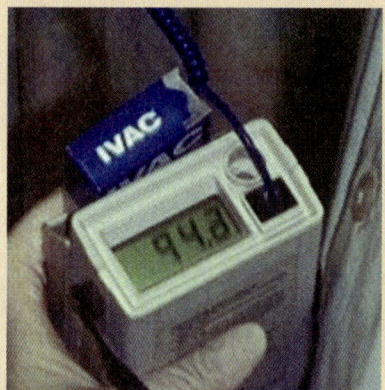

Figure 1-2-4 Listen for audible beep signal when temperature registers.

11. Instruct client to keep mouth closed around thermometer.

12. Thermometer will signal (beep) when a constant temperature registers (see Figure 1-2-4).

13. Read measurement on digital display of electronic thermometer. Push ejection button to discard disposable sheath into receptacle and return probe to storage well.

14. Inform client of temperature reading.

15. Remove gloves and wash hands.

16. Record reading according to agency policies.

17. Return electronic thermometer unit to charging base.

18. Wash hands.

11. Maintains thermometer in proper place and decreases amount of time required for an accurate reading.

12. Signal indicates final temperature reading.

13. Reduces transmission of microorganisms. Ensures that the electronic system is ready for next use.

14. Promotes client's participation in care.

15. Reduces transmission of microorganisms.

16. Accurate documentation by site allows for comparison of data.

17. Ensures charging base is plugged into electrical outlet and ready for next use.

18. Reduces transmission of microorganisms.

Tympanic Temperature: Infrared Thermometer

19. Repeat Actions 1–6.

20. Position client in Sims' or sitting position.

21. Remove probe from container and attach probe cover to tympanic thermometer unit (see Figure 1-2-5).

19. See Rationales 1–6.

20. Promotes access to ear.

21. Prevents contamination.

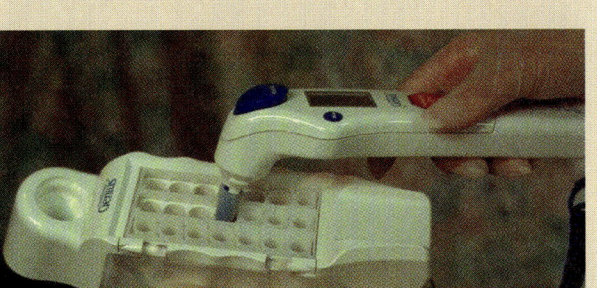

Figure 1-2-5 Attach disposable probe cover to unit.

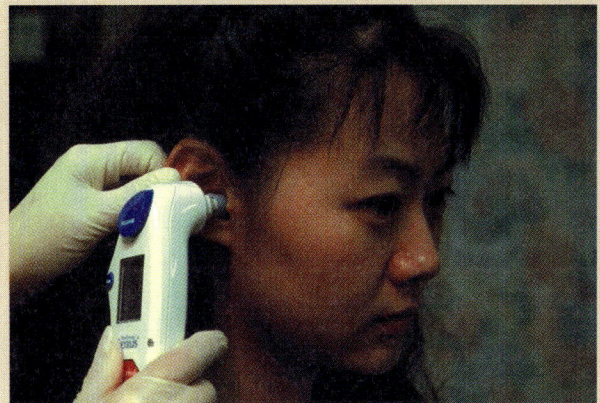

Figure 1-2-6 Insert temperature probe into ear canal.

22. Turn client's head to one side. For an adult, pull pinna upward and back; for a child, pull down and back. Gently insert probe with firm pressure into ear canal (see Figure 1-2-6).

23. Remove probe after the reading is displayed on digital unit (usually 2 seconds).

24. Remove probe cover and replace in storage container.

25. Return tympanic thermometer to storage unit.

26. Record reading according to agency policy.

27. Wash hands.

22. Provides access to ear canal. Gentle insertion prevents trauma to external canal. Firm pressure is needed to ensure probe will record an accurate temperature.

23. Reading is displayed within seconds.

24. Protects damage to the reusable probe.

25. Recharges batteries of unit for future use.

26. Promotes accurate documentation for data comparison.

27. Reduces transmission of microorganisms.

Using a "Tempa-Dot"

28. Repeat Actions 1–6.

29. Position the client in a sitting or lying position.

30. Prepare Tempa-Dot according to directions (see Figure 1-2-7).

28. See Rationales 1–6.

29. Promotes client's comfort, and promotes site access for all measurement.

30. Promotes accurate measurement and client safety.

continues

Using a "Tempa-Dot" continued

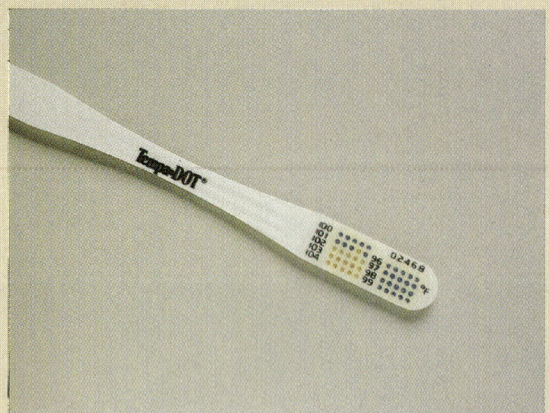

Figure 1-2-7 "Tempra-Dot" single-use disposable thermometer.

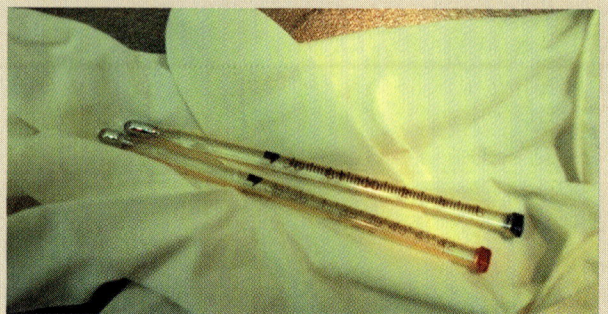

Figure 1-2-8 Oral (blue tip) and rectal (red tip) glass thermometers.

- Oral measurement: Place Tempa-Dot under tongue as far back as possible. Have client press tongue down on thermometer and keep mouth closed for 60 seconds. Remove thermometer, read the last blue dot; ignore any skipped dot.

- Axillary measurement: Place thermometer high in the armpit, vertical to the body, with dots against the torso. Lower client's arm to hold thermometer in place. Remove thermometer after 3 minutes.

31. Record temperature, indicate the method, and discard the thermometer.

31. Nursing documentation, practice clean technique.

32. Wash hands.

32. Reduces transmission of microorganisms.

33. Repeat Actions 1–6.

33. See Rationales 1–6.

34. Position the client in a sitting or lying position with the head of the bed elevated from 45 degrees to 60 degrees for measurement of all vital signs except those designated otherwise.

34. Promotes comfort, and improves site access for all measurements. Activity and movement can elevate heart and respiratory rates.

Oral Temperature: Glass Thermometer

35. Repeat steps 1–6, then select correct color tip of thermometer from client's bedside container (see Figure 1-2-8).

35. Identifies correct device; a blue tip usually denotes an oral thermometer.

36. Remove thermometer from storage container, hold at end away from bulb and cleanse under cool water.

36. Cleansing removes disinfectant, which can irritate oral mucosa. Cool water prevents expansion of the colored solution/mercury. Touching

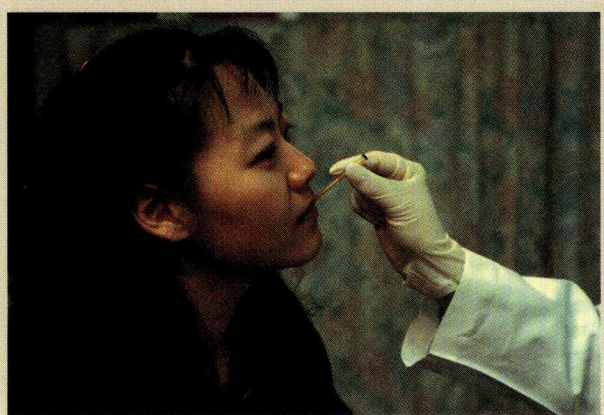

Figure 1-2-9 Place bulb of thermometer in the posterior sublingual pocket. Have client close mouth around thermometer.

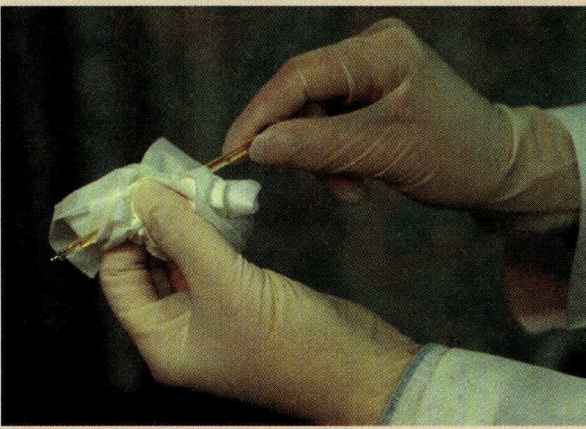

Figure 1-2-10 Wipe the thermometer with a tissue from bulb end to fingertips.

37. Use a tissue to dry thermometer from bulb's end toward fingertips.

38. Read thermometer by locating colored solution or mercury level. It should read 35.5°C (96°F).

39. If thermometer is not below normal body temperature reading, grasp thermometer with thumb and forefinger and shake vigorously by snapping the wrist in a downward motion to move mercury to a level below normal.

40. Place thermometer in client's mouth under the tongue and along the gumline to the posterior sublingual pocket. Instruct client to hold lips closed (see Figure 1-2-9).

41. Leave in place as specified by agency policy, usually 3–5 minutes.

42. Remove thermometer and wipe with a tissue away from fingers toward the bulb's end (see Figure 1-2-10).

43. Read at eye level and rotate slowly until mercury level is visualized.

the bulb will heat the solution and cause an inaccurate reading.

37. Wipe from area of least contamination to most contaminated area.

38. Thermometer must be below normal body temperature to ensure an accurate reading.

39. Shaking briskly lowers level of mercury in column. Because glass thermometers break easily, make sure that nothing in the environment comes in contact with the thermometer when shaking it.

40. Ensures contact with large blood vessels under the tongue. Prevents environmental air from coming in contact with the bulb.

41. Thermometer must stay in place long enough to ensure an accurate reading.

42. Mucus on thermometer may interfere with the effectiveness of the disinfectant solution. Wipe from area of least contamination to most contaminated area.

43. Ensures an accurate reading.

continues

Oral Temperature:
Glass Thermometer continued

44. Shake thermometer down, cleanse glass thermometer with soapy water, rinse under cold water, and return to storage container.

45. Remove and dispose of gloves in receptacle. Wash hands.

46. Record reading according to agency policy.

47. Wash hands.

Rectal Temperature

48. Repeat Actions 1–6.

49. Place client in the Sims' position with upper knee flexed. Adjust sheet to expose only anal area.

50. Place tissues in easy reach. Apply gloves.

51. Prepare the thermometer.

52. Lubricate tip of rectal thermometer or probe (a rectal thermometer usually has a red tip or cap).

53. With dominant hand, grasp thermometer. With other hand, separate buttocks to expose anus (see Figure 1-2-11).

44. Mechanical cleansing removes secretions that promote growth of microorganisms. Hot water may cause coagulation of secretions and cause expansion of mercury in the thermometer.

45. Reduces transmission of microorganisms.

46. Accurate documentation by site allows for comparison of data.

47. Reduces transmission of microorganisms.

48. See Rationales 1–6.

49. Proper positioning ensures visualization of anus. Flexing knee relaxes muscles for ease of insertion.

50. Tissue is needed to wipe anus after device is removed.

51. Ensures a smooth procedure and an accurate reading.

52. Promotes ease of insertion of thermometer or probe.

53. Aids in visualization of anus.

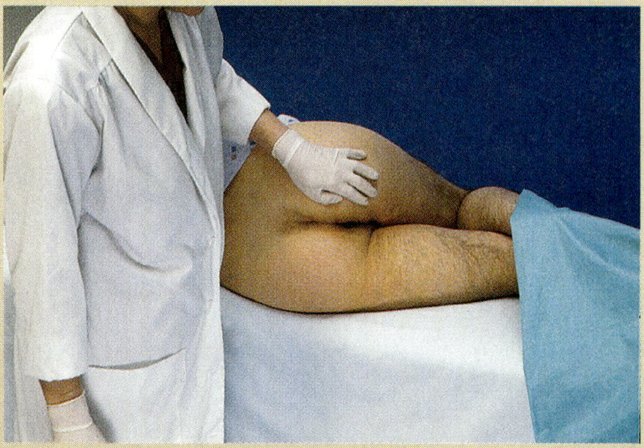

Figure 1-2-11 Preparation for the insertion of a rectal thermometer.

54. Instruct the client to take a deep breath. Insert the thermometer or probe gently into anus: infant, 1.2 cm (0.5 inches); adult, 3.5 cm (1.5 inches). If resistance is felt, do not force insertion.

54. Relaxes anal sphincter. Gentle insertion decreases discomfort to client and prevents trauma to mucous membranes.

55. Hold in place for 2 minutes.

55. Prevents trauma to mucosa and breakage of glass thermometer.

56. Wipe off secretions on the glass thermometer with a tissue. Dispose of tissue in a receptacle.

56. Removes secretions and fecal material for visualization of mercury level. Prevents transmission of microorganisms.

57. Read measurement and inform the client of the temperature reading.

57. Promotes client's participation in care.

58. While holding glass thermometer in one hand, use other hand to wipe anal area with tissue to remove lubricant or feces.
    Dispose of soiled tissue. Cover client.

58. Prevents contamination of clean objects with soiled thermometer, decreases skin irritation, and promotes client comfort. Prevents embarrassment.

59. Cleanse thermometer.

59. Reduces transmission of microorganisms.

60. Remove and dispose of gloves in receptacle. Wash hands.

60. Reduces transmission of microorganisms.

61. Record reading according to agency policy.

61. Accurate documentation by site allows for comparison of data.

Axillary Temperature

62. Repeat Actions 1–6.

62. See Rationales 1–6.

63. Remove client's arm and shoulder from one sleeve of gown. Avoid exposing chest.

63. Exposes axillary area.

64. Make sure axillary skin is dry; if necessary, pat dry.

64. Removes moisture and prevents a false low reading.

65. Prepare thermometer.

65. Ensures accurate use of thermometer.

66. Place thermometer or probe into center of axilla. Fold the client's upper arm straight down, and place arm across the client's chest.

66. Puts device in contact with axillary blood supply. Maintains the device in proper position.

67. Leave glass thermometer in place as specified by agency policy (usually 6–8 minutes). Leave an electronic thermometer in place until signal is heard.

67. Device must stay in place long enough to ensure an accurate reading. Signal indicates final temperature reading.

68. Remove and read thermometer.

68. Allows accurate reading of temperature.

69. Inform client of temperature reading.

69. Promotes client's participation in care.

continues

Axillary Temperature continued

70. Cleanse glass thermometer. Shake down thermometer, cleanse glass thermometer with soapy water, rinse under cold water, and return to storage container.	70. Prevents transmission of microorganisms and breakage of glass thermometer.
71. Assist the client with replacing the gown.	71. Promotes comfort.
72. Record reading according to agency policy.	72. Promotes accurate documentation for data comparison.
73. Wash hands.	73. Reduces transmission of microorganisms.

Disposable (Chemical Strip) Thermometer

74. Repeat Actions 1–6.	74. See Rationales 1–6.
75. Apply tape to appropriate skin area, usually forehead.	75. Tape must be in direct contact with the client's skin.
76. Observe tape for color changes.	76. Color indicates temperature reading (refer to the manufacturer's instructions).
77. Record reading and indicate method.	77. Promotes accurate documentation for data comparison.
78. Wash hands.	78. Reduces transmission of microorganisms.

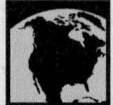

▶ **REAL WORLD ANECDOTES**

The visiting nurse is making a routine visit to John, a diabetic patient. John is a morbidly obese patient with diabetic leg ulcers. The physician's orders are for routine wet to dry dressing changes and blood glucose monitoring. While changing the dressing, the nurse notes that John says he is cold, yet his skin feels warm and looks flushed. His blood glucose is 310 mg/dl. There are no routine vital signs ordered, but the nurse feels that John may be seriously ill. John is chilling, and his teeth are chattering.

A glass thermometer is available, but the nurse feels John won't be able to hold it in his mouth firmly enough to get an accurate reading. Because he is obese, a rectal temperature would be difficult and time consuming. The nurse chooses to take an axillary temperature. The reading is 104°F. The nurse notifies John's doctor and John is admitted to the hospital with sepsis. In this case, "routine vital signs" became a critical assessment tool.

▶ **EVALUATION**

- Establish client's baseline temperature.
- Compare temperature with the client's baseline temperature.
- Evaluate the client's condition for trauma caused by the instrument.

▶ **DOCUMENTATION**

Vital Signs Flow Sheet

- Record the temperature measurement and site.
- Plot the temperature on a graph to identify patterns, or sudden elevations and drops (a condition known as spiking).

► VARIATIONS

Geriatric Variations:
- *Geriatric clients are more likely to be confused and unable to follow directions. It is especially important to be attentive and give clear, concise instructions when taking an oral temperature.*
- *Elderly clients may be more comfortable lying on their side with legs slightly flexed when taking a rectal temperature. Keep one hand on the thermometer and one hand on the client's hip so that you can detect if he/she starts to roll over. Place a pillow at the client's back for extra support, if needed.*
- *Baseline temperatures of elderly clients may be below the normal range; therefore increases should be compared with baseline.*

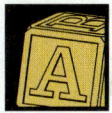

Pediatric Variations:
- *Infants and children often are not able to understand the nurse's instructions.*
- *Infants and children are often fearful of medical personnel and of the possibility of painful procedures. This may lead them to refuse to cooperate or to be combative.*
- *Infants and children may lie supine with knees flexed toward the abdomen as the nurse inserts the thermometer (see Figure 1-2-12).*
- *It may be more accurate to measure the pulse and respirations before the temperature if the child becomes agitated during temperature taking.*
- *Glass thermometers are not the best choice for young children. Tympanic or chemical strip thermometers are much less invasive, and less anxiety producing.*
- *When using the chemical strip thermometer, allow the child to place the strip and help you time the strip by holding your watch. Clean your watch before and after.*

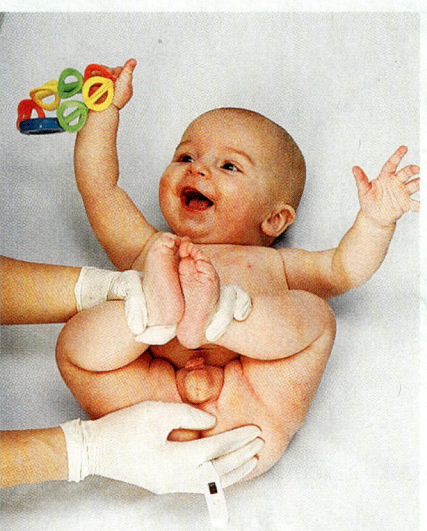

Figure 1-2-12 Taking a rectal temperature with infant in supine position.

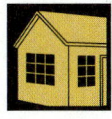

Home Care Variations:
- *Working equipment may not be available in the home care setting. The nurse should come prepared with working equipment, including a thermometer appropriate to the client.*
- *The temperature and ventilation of the room may affect the client's temperature.*
- *Remember to bring the best type of thermometer for the client with you for your home health visit.*

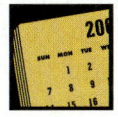

Long-Term-Care Variation:
- *Long-term-care clients more often have physical limitations that must be considered when choosing the route to use in measuring the internal temperature. When considering route in a long-term-care client, consider the possibility of a stoma where the rectum has been surgically closed or perhaps severe contractures that would make client positioning and cooperation difficult and painful.*

► COMMON ERRORS

Possible Error:

You are in a hurry and left the oral thermometer in the client's mouth for only 2 minutes.

Prevention:

Use the equipment and its signals such as the beep of the electronic thermometer. Know the recommended length of time to leave a glass thermometer in place for an oral, axillary, and rectal temperature.

Take the temperature again and observe the recommended time.

Medication Administration Record

- Record doses of antipyretic (fever-reducing) medications and temperature reading.

Nurses' Notes

- Record response to antipyretic medications.

► CRITICAL THINKING SKILL

Introduction

Use good judgment when choosing the site used to measure a temperature. An accurate reading requires use of all the assessment skills described.

Possible Scenario

You are assigned to work in the newborn nursery this evening. You are assessing a newborn. Using your nursing judgment you must determine the best method to evaluate the baby's internal temperature. Because you do not want to hurt the baby, you choose a glass thermometer and place it under the baby's arm.

Possible Outcome

Because this is the first temperature reading done on this client, it is an inaccurately low reading and fails to detect a problem. It also creates an incorrect baseline for future comparisons.

Prevention

You should realize that there are a number of factors that must enter into this decision. An oral temperature is contraindicated in newborns because they cannot follow instructions to keep their mouths closed and not bite the thermometer. An axillary temperature would be safe, but would yield the least accurate reading. A tympanic reading would be less invasive than the rectal temperature and more comfortable for the infant, but it is less accurate in infants. The rectal temperature is the preferred method for assessing newborn temperatures. Not only is it the most accurate method available to nurses but it also gives the nurse an opportunity to assess the structure and patency of the baby's anus, an important part of the newborn physical exam. So you should use the rectal thermometer to obtain an accurate reading.

► NURSING TIPS

- For the best comparison of the client's longitudinal temperature readings, the temperature should be taken at the same time every day using the same method.
- After giving antipyretic medication to a client, a temperature measurement should be taken 30 minutes after the intervention and then every 2 to 4 hours. Nursing intervention policy may vary across institutions.
- Oral, rectal, and tympanic temperature measurements are higher than axillary measurements because the measuring device is in contact with the mucous membrane.
- Rectal measurements are higher than oral measurements because of the seal created by the anal

sphincter, which decreases contact with environmental influences.
- Avoid rinsing a glass thermometer in hot water. Hot water can cause the thermometer to expand and break.
- The client should not insert a rectal thermometer without assistance. Inappropriate application can cause tissue trauma.
- Continuous temperature monitoring can be done using a rectal probe, or a special urinary catheter.
- When checking the chart for trends in temperature, make sure the same measurement device was used. As noted in Table 1-2-1, the normal range varies according to the device used.

Table 1-2-1 Advantages and Disadvantages of Four Routes for Body Temperature Measurement

ROUTE	NORMAL RANGE	ADVANTAGES	DISADVANTAGES
ORAL Average 37.0°C or 98.6°F	36.0°–38.0°C 96.8°–100.4°F	Convenient; accessible	**Safety:** Glass thermometers with colored solution/mercury can be bitten and broken, causing patient injury. Patients need to be alert and cooperative and cognitively capable of following instructions for safe use. **Physical abilities:** Patients need to be able to breathe through the nose, and be without oral pathology or recent oral surgery; route not applicable for comatose or confused patients. **Accuracy:** Oxygen therapy by mask or ingestion of hot or cold drinks immediately before oral temperature measurement, affects accuracy of the reading.
RECTAL Average 0.7°C or 0.4°F higher than oral	36.7°–38.7°C 100.4°–100.8°F	Considered most accurate	**Safety:** Contraindicated following rectal surgery. Risk of rectal Valsalva's perforation in children less than 2 years of age. Risk of stimulating Valsalva's maneuver in cardiac patients. **Physical aspects:** Invasive and uncomfortable.
AXILLARY Average 0.6°C or 1°F lower than oral	35.4°–37.4°C 95.8°–99.4°F	Safe; noninvasive	**Accuracy:** Glass thermometer must be left in place for 5 minutes to obtain accurate measurement. Placement and position of thermometer tip affect reading.
TYMPANIC Calibrated to oral or rectal scales	See oral or rectal	Convenient; fast; safe; noninvasive. Does not require contact with any mucous membrane.	**Accuracy:** Research is inconclusive as to accuracy of readings and correlations with other body temperature measurements. Technique affects reading. Tympanic membrane is thought to reflect the core temperature.

▶ SPECIAL CONSIDERATIONS

- *Since mercury is hepatotoxic, alternative thermometers should be used. If your facility uses colored solution/mercury thermometers, you must know the policy for management of broken thermometers as well as disposal of thermometers.*
- *If your client has a seizure disorder or is a mouth breather, you should avoid using a glass, oral thermometer for temperature measurement.*
- *Taking a rectal temperature should be avoided when a client is receiving medication rectally when diarrhea is present.*

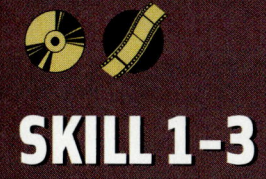

SKILL 1-3

Taking a Pulse

Karrin Johnson, RN, and Hsin-Yi (Jean) Tang, RN, PhD

KEY TERMS

Apical pulse
Bradycardia
Pedal pulse
Popliteal pulse
Pulse deficit
Radial pulse
Tachycardia
Temporal pulse

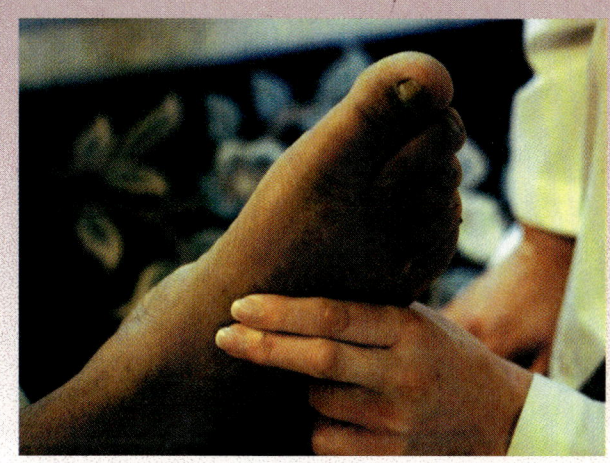

▶ OVERVIEW OF THE SKILL

Pulse assessment is the measurement of a pressure pulsation created when the heart contracts and ejects blood into the aorta. The amplitude of the pulse reflects the stroke volume with each ejection. Assessment of pulse characteristics provides clinical data regarding the heart's pumping action and the adequacy of peripheral artery blood flow. The radial pulse is most often used for basic assessment; however, other site areas are used in total assessment and when specific areas of circulation are to be determined.

▶ PULSE-TAKING TECHNIQUES

Palpation

- Palpation of a pulse involves the index and middle fingers of one hand. Start with gentle pressure to locate the strongest pulsation, and then use firmer palpation for the counting. When counting, also assess the rhythm and quality of the pulse. Measure the pulse for 30 and 60 seconds, and then multiply the counts if need be to obtain the one-minute reading.

Auscultation

- Auscultation is usually used to assess the apical pulse. The apical pulse is the most accurate pulse, especially when the peripheral pulse is difficult to locate. Auscultation requires the stethoscope. The stethoscope should be equipped with a bell and a diaphragm. The diaphragm side is normally used for low-pitch sound, such as like normal heart sound, bowel sound, or breath sound; the bell side is used for high-pitch sound, such as murmur and abnormal heart sound.

Doppler

- An ultrasonic Doppler device is usually used when the pulse cannot be detected by palpation. The Doppler can detect the peripheral pulses in situations such as cardiopulmonary collapse, in obese clients, infants with small arms, or clients with edema in which palpation of the pulse is difficult.
- A vendor-recommended conductive gel should be applied to the skin as a coupling medium for ultrasound transmission. The transmitting device (probe) is then placed over the artery to be assessed. The Doppler usually is equipped with both high- and low-frequency probes. High-frequency (8–10 Hz) probe is usually used on the surface vessel sites. Low-frequency (2–3 Hz) probe often is used for deeper sites, such as obstetrical assessment.
- The sounds can be amplified and heard through an earpiece or speaker attached to the device, assessing with low volume initially. Tilt the back of the probe toward the hand at an angle of about 45 degrees.

Search the area of the assessed artery, and tilt the probe for best Doppler sounds. Adjust the sound volume control to a comfort level for counting.

▶ ASSESSMENT

1. Assess client for need to monitor pulse **because certain diseases or conditions, such as history of heart disease or cardiac dysrhythmias, chest pain, invasive cardiovascular diagnostic tests, infusion of large volume of IV fluids, or hemorrhage, can cause an increased risk for alterations in pulse.**
2. Assess the pulse for rate, amplitude, contour, and regularity.
3. Assess for signs and symptoms of cardiovascular alterations, such as dyspnea, chest pain, orthopnea, syncope, palpitations, edema of extremities, cyanosis or fatigue, **because these signs may indicate a deficit in cardiac or vascular function.**
4. Assess client for factors that may affect the character of the pulse, such as age, medications, exercise, change in position, or fever. **This enables the nurse to accurately assess for the significance of an alteration in pulse.**
5. Assess for the appropriate site for measuring pulse **so that the pulse will be accurate.**
6. Assess the baseline heart rate and rhythm in the client's chart **in order to compare it with the current measurement.**
7. Assess circulatory status by using appropriate site (Table 1-3-1) since pulses may be affected by surgery, medical condition, arterial blood draws, or poor circulation.

▶ DIAGNOSIS

- Decreased Cardiac Output, due to alteration in the rate and rhythm of pulse.
- Ineffective Cardiopulmonary Tissue Perfusion.

▶ PLANNING

Expected Outcomes:

1. Pulse rate, quality, rhythm, and volume will be within normal range for the client's age group.

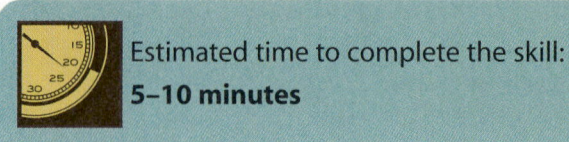
Estimated time to complete the skill: 5–10 minutes

2. The client will be comfortable with the procedure and demonstrate an understanding regarding its importance.

Equipment Needed (see Figure 1-3-1):
- Watch with a second hand
- Stethoscope
- Alcohol swab
- Gloves

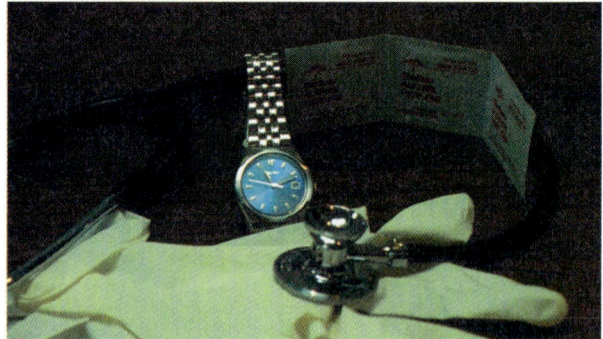

Figure 1-3-1 A watch with a second hand is used to count pulse. Use a stethoscope to assess apical pulse. Gloves and alcohol swabs reduce the transmission of microorganisms.

▶ CLIENT EDUCATION NEEDED

1. Ask the client to relax and sit or lie quietly while you take the pulse rate.
2. Explain the normal pulse range when telling the client what the pulse rate is. This eases the client's concerns regarding whether or not the rate is "normal."
3. If the client is taking any medications that affect pulse rate, this is a good time to review the name and purpose of this medication.
4. If taking a pulse at a site other than radial, explain to the client the reason for using an alternate site.
5. Have the client breathe normally through the nose, especially if taking an apical pulse. Breathing through the nose decreases breath sounds, making the heart sounds easier to hear.

Table 1-3-1 Pulse Point Assessment

PULSE POINT		ASSESSMENT CRITERIA
SITES OF THE PULSATION MEASUREMENT		
SITE	**LOCATION**	
1. Temporal	Over the temporal bone, lateral to the eye, upper to the ear	Accessible; used routinely for infants and when radial is inaccessible
2. Carotid	Bilateral, under the lower jaw, beneath the sternomastoid muscles. Carotid pulse best represents the aortic pulse for its close location to the central circulation. Palpation of the carotid artery on the neck may cause stimulation of the carotid sinus and result in decrease of down of the pulse rate	Accessible; used routinely for infants and during shock or cardiac arrest when other peripheral pulses are too weak to palpate; also used to assess cranial circulation
3. Apical	Left ventricle, fourth to fifth intercostal space, on the midclavicular line	Used to auscultate heart sounds and assess apical-radial deficit
4. Brachial	Inner side between the groove of bicep and tricep muscles at the antecubital fossa	Used in cardiac arrest for infants, to assess lower arm circulation, and to auscultate blood pressure
5. Radial	On the thumb side, inner aspect of the wrist	Accessible; used routinely in adults to assess character of peripheral pulse
6. Ulnar	On the little finger side, outer aspect of the wrist	Used to assess circulation to ulnar side of hand and to perform the Allen test
7. Femoral	Below the inguinal ligament, in the anterior medial aspect of the thigh, midway to the anterior-superior iliac spine and symphysis pubis	Used to assess circulation to legs and during cardiac arrest
8. Popliteal	Behind the knee. Medial or lateral to the popliteal fossa	Used to assess circulation to legs and to auscultate leg blood pressure
9. Posterior Tibial	Inner side of the ankle, between the Achilles' tendon and tibia	Used to assess circulation to feet
10. Pedal/Dorsal Pedal	Lateral to the extension tendon, from the great toe toward the ankle	Used to assess circulation to feet

▶ DELEGATION TIPS

The radial pulse assessment is often delegated to trained ancillary personnel; however, the nurse is responsible for knowing the results. Assessment of the apical pulse may be delegated to specially prepared staff. The assessment of peripheral circulation is delegated after proper training in the monitoring of peripheral sites, for the presence of abnormal color, motion, or sensation in the extremity. The absence of pulses must be immediately reported for further assessment by the nurse, and the nurse is responsible for reviewing the data collected in a timely manner and revalidating the results, if indicated. The agency's policy should clearly indicate the training and validation requirements before the nurse delegates the monitoring of apical pulses and peripheral vascular assessments on stable clients. These tasks should not be delegated if the client is unstable.

IMPLEMENTATION—ACTION/RATIONALE

ACTION	RATIONALE
Taking a Radial (Wrist) Pulse	
1. Wash hands.	1. Reduces transmission of microorganisms.
2. Inform client of the site(s) at which you will measure pulse.	2. Encourages participation and allays anxiety.
3. Flex client's elbow and place lower part of arm across chest.	3. Maintains wrist in full extension and exposes artery for palpation. Placing client's hand over chest will facilitate later respiratory assessment without undue attention to your action. (It is difficult for any person to maintain a normal breathing pattern when someone is observing and measuring.)
4. Support client's wrist by grasping outer aspect with thumb.	4. Stabilizes wrist and allows for pressure to be exerted.
5. Place your index and middle fingers on inner aspect of client's wrist over the radial artery and apply light but firm pressure until pulse is palpated (see Figure 1-3-2).	5. Fingertips are sensitive, facilitating palpation of pulsating pulse. The nurse may feel her own pulse if palpating with thumb. Applying light pressure prevents occlusion of blood flow and pulsation.

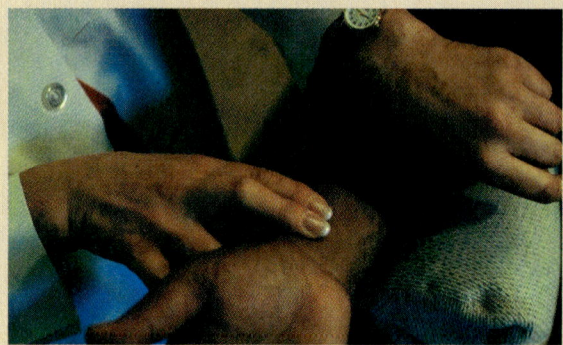

Figure 1-3-2 Place index and middle fingers over radial artery.

6. Identify pulse rhythm.	6. Palpate pulse until rhythm is determined. Describe as regular or irregular.
7. Determine pulse volume.	7. Quality of pulse strength is an indication of stroke volume. Describe as normal, weak, strong, or bounding.
8. Count pulse rate by using second hand on watch (see Figure 1-3-3). For a regular rhythm, count number of beats for 30 seconds and multiply by 2.	8. An irregular rhythm requires a full minute of assessment to identify the number of inefficient cardiac contractions that fail to transmit a pulsation, referred to as a "skipped" or irregular beat.

For an irregular rhythm, count number of beats for a full minute, noting number of irregular beats.

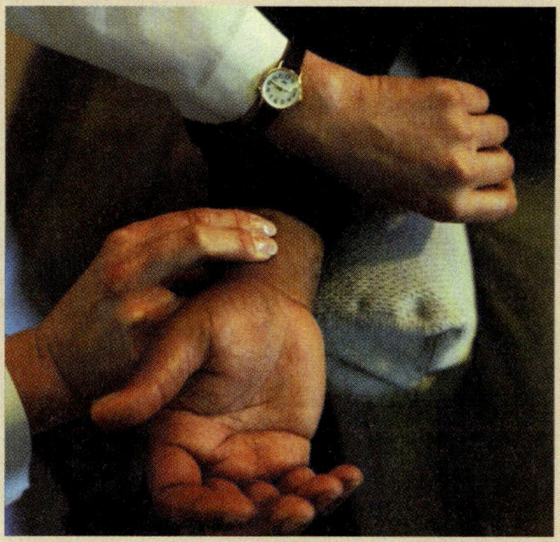

Figure 1-3-3 Count pulse rate for 30 seconds. Multiply by 2.

Taking an Apical Pulse

9. Wash hands.

10. Raise client's gown to expose sternum and left side of chest.

11. Cleanse earpiece and diaphragm of stethoscope with an alcohol swab.

12. Put stethoscope around your neck.

13. Locate apex of heart:
    - With client lying on left side, locate suprasternal notch.
    - Palpate second intercostal space to left of sternum.
    - Place index finger in intercostal space, counting downward until fifth intercostal space is located.
    - Move index finger along fourth intercostal space left of the sternal border and to the fifth intercostal space, left of the midclavicular line to palpate the point of maximal impulse (PMI) (see Figure 1-3-4).
    - Keep index finger of nondominant hand on the PMI.

14. Inform client that you are going to listen to his heart. Instruct client to remain silent.

15. With dominant hand, put earpiece of the stethoscope in your ears and grasp diaphragm of the stethoscope in palm of your hand for 5–10 seconds.

9. Reduces transmission of microorganisms.

10. Allows access to client's chest for proper placement of stethoscope.

11. Decreases transmission of microorganisms from one practitioner to another (earpiece) and from one client to another (diaphragm).

12. Ensures stethoscope is nearby for frequent use.

13. Identification of landmarks facilitates correct placement of the stethoscope at the fifth intercostal space in order to hear point of maximal impulse.
    - Ensures correct placement of stethoscope.

14. Elicits client support. Stethoscope amplifies noise.

15. Dominant hand facilitates psychomotor dexterity for placement of earpiece with one hand. Heat warms metal or plastic diaphragm and prevents startling client.

continues

Taking an Apical Pulse *continued*

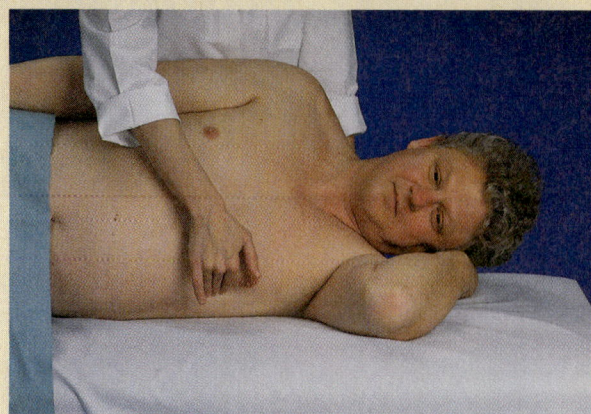

Figure 1-3-4 Palpating the apical pulse.

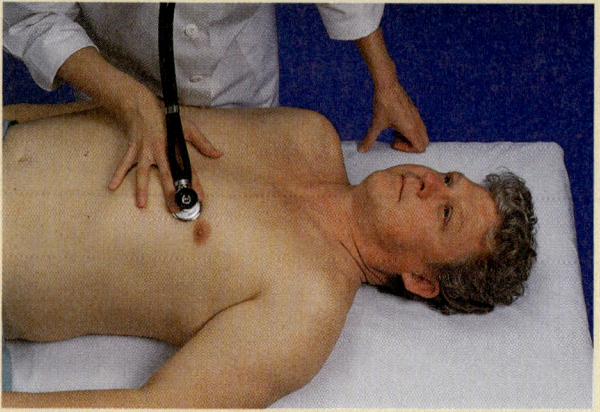

Figure 1-3-5 Place diaphragm of stethoscope over the PMI to hear the heart rate.

16. Place diaphragm of stethoscope over the PMI and auscultate for sounds S_1 and S_2 to hear lub-dub sound (see Figure 1-3-5).

17. Note regularity of rhythm.

18. Start to count while looking at second hand of watch. Count lub-dub sound as one beat:
    - For a regular rhythm, count rate for 30 seconds and multiply by 2.
    - For an irregular rhythm, count rate for a full minute, noting number of irregular beats.

19. Share your findings with client.

20. Record by site the rate, rhythm, and, if applicable, number of irregular beats.

21. Wash hands.

16. Movement of blood through the heart valves creates S_1 and S_2 sounds. Listen for a regular rhythm (heartbeats are evenly spaced) before counting.

17. Establishment of a rhythmic pattern determines length of time to count the heartbeats to ensure accurate measurement.

18. Ensures sufficient time to count irregular beats.

19. Promotes client participation in care.

20. Record rate and characteristics at bedside to ensure accurate documentation.

21. Reduces transmission of microorganisms.

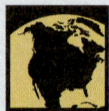 ▶ **REAL WORLD ANECDOTES**

A 74-year-old male presents to the emergency room complaining of pain in his chest. While taking routine vital signs, the nurse notes that both his apical and radial pulse are 44 beats per minute. The nurse considers the possibility that heart conductivity problems may be causing this low rate.

The client's EKG on the cardiac monitor appears normal. While taking a more complete history, the client states that he is a marathon runner and he takes his pulse rate himself daily as part of his training. The client notes that his pulse rate normally runs quite low. He also states that he just ate a large, spicy meal, an alternative explanation for his chest pain, which needs further assessment. The nurse makes a mental note not to jump to conclusions without a thorough history and physical.

SKILL 1-3 Taking a Pulse

Table 1-3-2 Scales for Measuring Pulse Volume

3-POINT SCALE		4-POINT SCALE	
SCALE	DESCRIPTION OF PULSE	SCALE	DESCRIPTION OF PULSE
0	Absent	0	Absent
1+	Thready/weak	1+	Thready/weak
2+	Normal	2+	Normal
3+	Bounding	3+	Increased
		4+	Bounding

▶ EVALUATION

- Compare client's pulse with baseline rate, amplitude, and rhythm to detect any changes (see Table 1-3-2).
- If pulse is irregular or abnormal, ask another nurse to check the pulse and then report to physician or qualified practitioner.
- Evaluate pulse site (see Table 1-3-1) as required by client's condition and compare bilateral pulses. Example: For clients with poor peripheral circulation in the lower extremities, compare both pedal/dorsal or both posterior tibial pulses.

▶ DOCUMENTATION

Nurses' Notes and/or Flow Sheet

- Pulse rate
- Observations regarding regularity, volume, or rate
- New irregularities in pulse reported to the patient's physician or qualified practitioner

▶ CRITICAL THINKING SKILL

Introduction

A pulse deficit is a condition where the apical pulse is greater than the radial pulse rate. A pulse deficit exists when the heart is not ejecting enough blood volume to initiate a peripheral pulse wave. If left untreated, this can lead to serious complications. Check for a pulse deficit if the amplitude of pulsation is not the same with each beat. Check an apical pulse and assess any EKG changes. Because a client may not have a strong stroke volume with each beat, further cardiac assessment is needed.

Possible Scenario

You are taking a radial pulse on a client who was admitted to the coronary care unit. The client's pulse volume is weak and thready. The radial pulse is slow and irregular. You are concerned and take an apical pulse as well. His apical pulse is faster than his radial pulse and is regular. You check the nursing record, but see no mention of this finding.

Possible Outcome

You chart your findings and report them immediately to the client's physician. He confirms your finding of a pulse deficit and orders immediate intervention to increase this client's cardiac ejection volumes.

Prevention

Remember that the nature of the pulse volume, rate, and regularity is a valuable tool in assessing a client's overall health and in diagnosing disease states.

▶ VARIATIONS

Geriatric Variations:
- Tremors in geriatric clients can interfere with evaluating the radial pulse accurately.
- An apical or carotid pulse might be the better option in older clients.

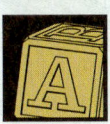

Pediatric Variations:
- Radial pulses on infants are not reliable because of the small size of the client and the rapid heart rate normal in infants. A temporal or apical pulse is preferable.
- The PMI in an infant is usually located at the third to fourth intercostal space near the sternum.

▶ VARIATIONS continued

- *A child may be more comfortable sitting on his mother's lap while having his pulse assessed.*
- *A curious child may be more cooperative if he can listen to his own heart with a stethoscope.*

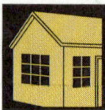

Home Care Variations:
- *The home care environment can be distracting for the nurse and the client. The television and loud music can make it difficult to hear an apical pulse and can artificially elevate the client's pulse rate.*
- *Be sure that the client is sitting or lying quietly before taking the pulse.*
- *Clients can be taught to assess their own pulse, especially when taking cardiac medications.*

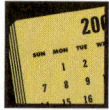

Long-Term-Care Variation:
- *The relative immobility of most long-term-care clients puts them at risk of decreased peripheral circulation. Pedal pulses are an important part of the nursing examination in long-term-care clients.*

▶ COMMON ERRORS

Possible Error:

You count the pulse of a client with a cardiac arrhythmia for 15 seconds and then multiply the rate by 4 to obtain a one-minute pulse rate.

Prevention:

Count the heart rate for at least 30 seconds to increase the probability of noting irregularities. Some irregularities do not occur in intervals of less than 15 seconds. Occasional premature beats or brief runs of supraventricular tachycardia can be missed.

Count the pulse for a full minute, noting the regularity or irregularity of the beats.

▶ NURSING TIPS

- Warm the bell of the stethoscope with your hands prior to placing it on the client's chest.
- Take a carotid pulse on only one side of the neck at a time in order to prevent cerebral blood flow impairment (see Figure 1-3-6).
- When taking pedal pulses, a firm touch is generally preferable to reduce any tickling sensations.
- A Doppler device may be necessary to detect a pulse on elderly or obese clients (see Figure 1-3-7).

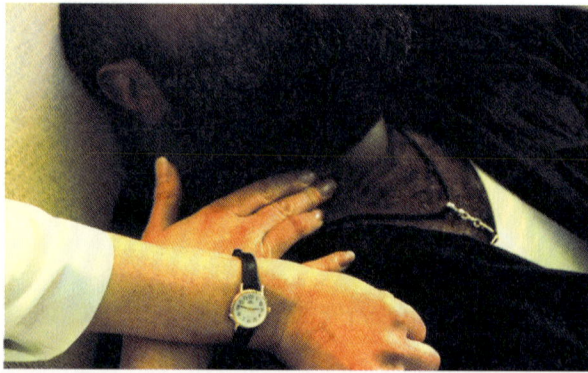

Figure 1-3-6 Take a carotid pulse on only one side of the neck at a time.

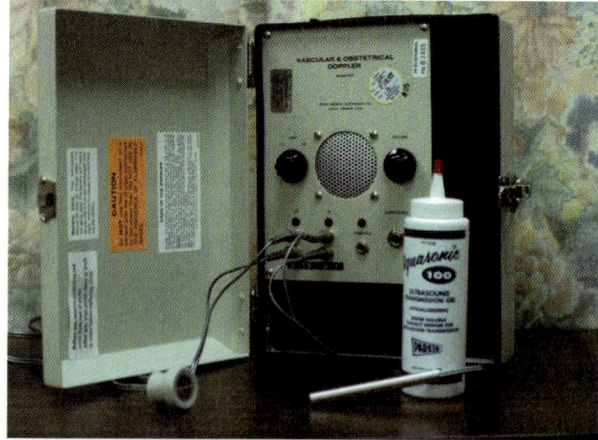

Figure 1-3-7 A vascular Doppler device is used to detect pulses in elderly or obese patients.

▶ SPECIAL CONSIDERATIONS

- *Never use the thumb to obtain a pulse because you may sense a beat from your own digital artery that can alter an accurate reading.*
- *When using a Doppler to obtain a fetal heart beat check the mother's pulse to ensure the beat heard is indeed that of the fetus.*
- *When preparing a client for surgery related to venous insufficiency of the lower extremities (i.e., femoral-popliteal bypass), it is essential to mark the pedal pulses with an "X." This facilitates locating the pulse during surgery, to confirm circulation for the surgeon.*

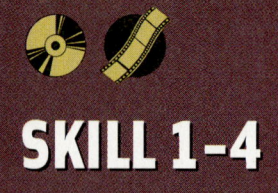

SKILL 1-4: Counting Respirations

Karrin Johnson, RN and Gaylene Bouska Altman, RN, PhD

KEY TERMS

Apnea
Bradypnea
Cheyne-Stokes respirations
Cyanosis
Diaphragm
Dyspnea
Eupnea
Hyperpnea
Hyperventilation
Hypoventilation
Kussmaul's respirations
Orthopnea
Pleura
Tachypnea

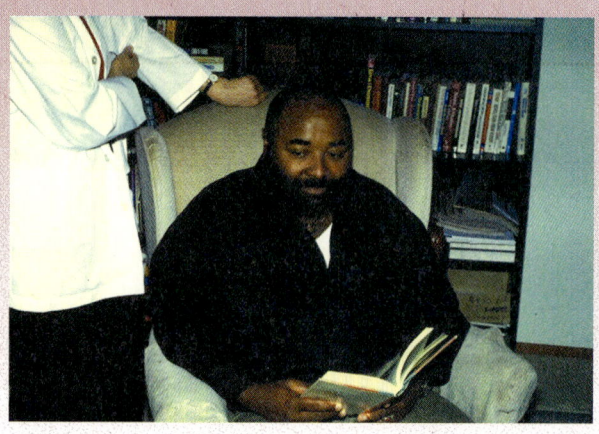

▶ OVERVIEW OF THE SKILL

Respiratory assessment is the measurement of the breathing pattern. Assessment of respirations provides clinical data regarding the pH of arterial blood.

Normal breathing is slightly observable, effortless, quiet, automatic, and regular. It can be assessed by observing chest wall expansion and bilateral symmetrical movement of the thorax or by placing the back of the hand next to the client's nose and mouth to feel the expired air.

When assessing respiration, ascertain the rate, depth, and rhythm of ventilatory movement. The nurse should assess the rate by counting the number of breaths taken per minute. Note the depth and rhythm of ventilatory movements by observing for the normal thoracic and abdominal movements and symmetry in chest wall movement. Normal respirations are characterized by a rate ranging from 12 to 20 breaths per minute.

One inspiration and expiration cycle is counted as one breath. The nurse can observe the rise and fall of the chest wall and count the rate by placing the hand lightly on the chest to feel it rise and fall. Count the number of respirations for a 30-second interval and multiply by 2 if respirations are regular and even. If the client is experiencing any respiratory difficulty, count the rate for a full minute.

When the chest wall moves, so do the lungs, because the lungs are attached to the inner wall of the thoracic cavity by the outer layer of the pleura (lining of the chest cavity). The movement of the chest wall should be even and regular, without noise and effort. On inspiration the chest changes shape and expands as the rib cage is raised and the diaphragm is lowered. Before inspiration, the pressure inside the chest cavity is negative (-4.5 to -9.0 mm Hg below atmospheric pressure). Air flows along the concentration gradient from a higher atmospheric pressure to the lower intrathoracic pressure.

The opposite action occurs with expiration. The muscles relax, causing the rib cage to lower, and the diaphragm to rise, compressing the chest. Intrathoracic pressure decreases to -3 to -6 mm Hg to allow the air to escape into the atmosphere.

Different respiratory wave patterns are characterized by their rate, rhythm, and depth. Eupnea refers to easy respirations with a normal rate of breaths per minute that are age specific. Bradypnea is a respiratory rate of 10 or fewer breaths per minute. Hypoventilation is characterized by shallow respirations. Tachypnea is a respiratory rate greater than 24 breaths per minute. Hyperventilation is characterized by deep, rapid respirations. Hyperpnea occurs with exercise when respirations are increased in depth and rate. Sighing is a protective physiologic mechanism for expanding small airways not used with normal breathing.

The nurse can also observe alterations in the movement of the chest wall: costal (thoracic) breathing occurs when the external intercostal muscles and the other accessory muscles are used to move the chest

SKILL 1-4 Counting Respirations

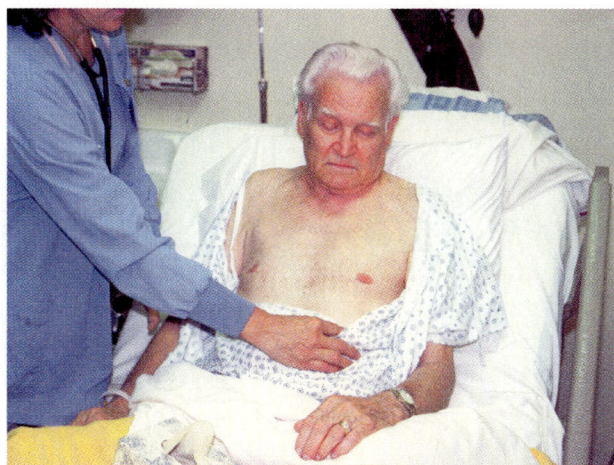

Figure 1-4-1 Observe the movement of the chest wall and assess the quality and depth of respiration. Place your hand below the diaphragm to feel if the patient is using his diaphragm instead of expanding his chest wall to bring air into the lungs.

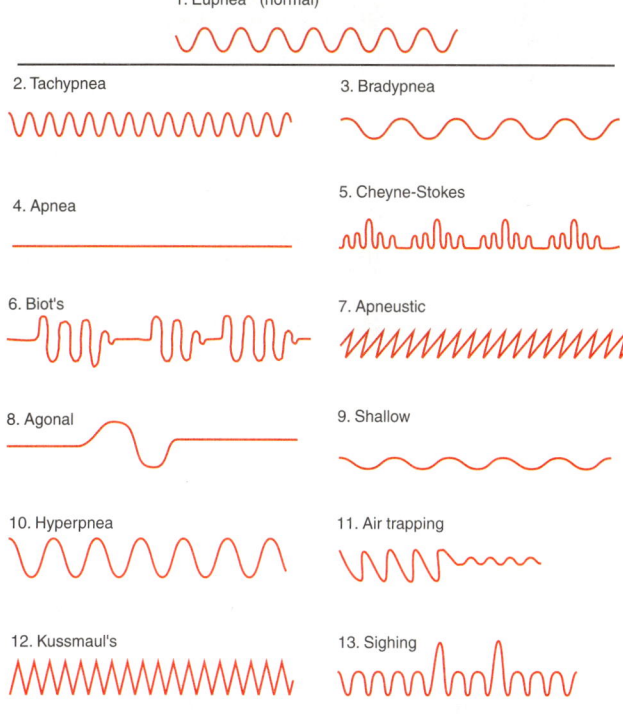

Figure 1-4-2 Normal and abnormal respiratory patterns.

upward and outward; diaphragmatic (abdominal) breathing occurs when the diaphragm contracts and relaxes as observed by movement of the abdomen. Dyspnea refers to difficulty in breathing as observed by labored or forced respirations through the use of accessory muscles in the chest and neck to breathe. Dyspneic clients are acutely aware of their respirations and complain of shortness of breath (see Figure 1-4-1).

Respiratory alterations may cause changes in skin color as observed by a bluish appearance of the nailbeds, lips, and skin. The bluish color (cyanosis) results from reduced oxygen levels in the arterial blood. Changes in the level of consciousness (restlessness, anxiety, and dyspnea) may also occur with decreased oxygen levels. Clients with orthopnea may assume a forward-leaning position or may have to stand to increase the expansion capacity of the lungs.

Metabolic alterations such as diabetic ketoacidosis can cause Kussmaul's respirations, which are abnormally deep but regular.

Apnea is the cessation of breathing for several seconds. Persistent apnea is called respiratory arrest. Irregular rhythm with alternating periods of apnea and hyperventilation is called Cheyne-Stokes respirations

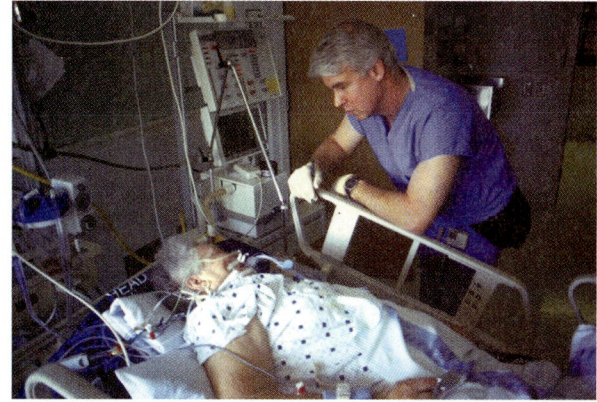

Figure 1-4-3 When assessing respirations, observe skin color and level of consciousness as well as respiratory rate and rhythm.

(see Figure 1-4-2). The cycle begins with slow, shallow breaths that gradually increase to abnormally deep and rapid respirations, which then gradually slow and return to shallow breathing followed by apnea. This is common in dying patients (see Figure 1-4-3).

▶ ASSESSMENT

1. Assess the movement of client's chest wall **to see if it is equal bilaterally, if the movement is labored, or if the client is using accessory muscles to breathe.**
2. Assess the rate of respirations **to identify slow, rapid, or irregular respirations or even periods of apnea.**
3. Assess the depth of the client's breaths in order **to monitor shallow, deep, or uneven respirations. Think if there is something influencing the client's respirations. Is he/she in pain, frightened, talking, smoking?**

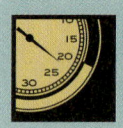 Estimated time to complete the skill: **3 minutes**

4. Assess for risk factors such as fever, pain, anxiety, diseases, or trauma to the chest wall **that may alter the respirations because certain conditions may cause increased risk of alterations in respirations.**
5. Assess for factors that normally influence respirations such as age, exercise, anxiety, pain, smoking, medications, or postural changes **so that an accurate assessment can be made.**

▶ DIAGNOSIS

- Impaired Gas Exchange.
- Impaired Spontaneous Ventilation.
- Ineffective Airway Clearance.
- Ineffective Breathing Pattern.

▶ PLANNING

Expected Outcomes:

1. An accurate evaluation of a client's respiratory rate and character will be obtained.
2. The respiratory rate and character will be normal.

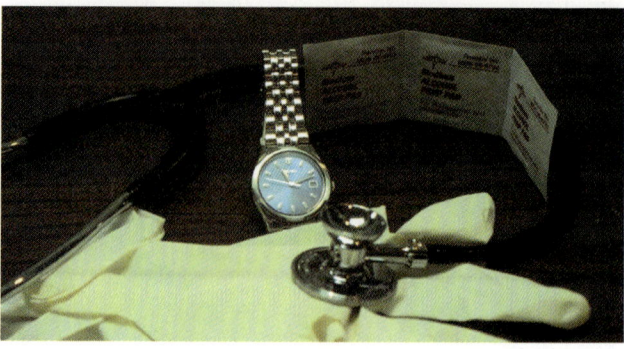

Figure 1-4-4 A watch with a second hand is used to assess respirations.

Equipment Needed (see Figure 1-4-4):

- Watch with a second hand
- Stethoscope if needed

▶ CLIENT EDUCATION NEEDED

1. Instruct the client about the reason for assessing respirations.
2. Teach the caregiver to count respirations while the client is not aware.
3. Instruct the caregiver to contact the nurse if there is an alteration in the client's respirations.
4. Clients should be taught to notify their caregiver or nurse when they feel a change in their respirations.
5. Clients who have decreased ventilation may benefit from being taught deep-breathing and coughing techniques.

▶ DELEGATION TIPS

The skill of respiratory rate measurement is often delegated to ancillary personnel; however, the nurse is responsible for this information and appropriate action. Respiration counts over 30 (adult) or 60 (child) should immediately be reported to the nurse for further assessment.

IMPLEMENTATION—ACTION/RATIONALE

ACTION	RATIONALE
1. Wash hands.	1. Reduces transmission of microorganisms.
2. Be sure chest movement is visible. Client may need to remove heavy clothing.	2. Facilitates observation of chest wall and abdominal movements.

SKILL 1-4 Counting Respirations

3. Observe one complete respiratory cycle. If it is easier, place the client's hand across his abdomen and your hand over the client's wrist.

4. Start counting with first inspiration while looking at the second hand of a watch (see Figure 1-4-5).
   - Infants and children: count a full minute.
   - Adults: count for 30 seconds and multiply by 2. If an irregular rate or rhythm is present, count for one full minute.

5. Observe character of respirations:
   - Depth of respirations by degree of chest wall movement (shallow, normal, or deep)
   - Rhythm of cycle (regular or interrupted)

6. Replace client's gown if needed.

7. Record rate and character of respirations.

8. Wash hands.

3. Helps determine what constitutes a breath. Helps to determine what to count. Hand rises and falls with inspiration and expiration.

4. Respiratory rate is one complete cycle (inspiration and expiration).
   - Infants and children usually have an irregular rate.

5. Reveals volume of air movement into and out of the lungs.

6. Prevents embarrassment and chilling.

7. Record rate and characteristics at bedside to ensure accurate documentation.

8. Reduces transmission of microorganisms.

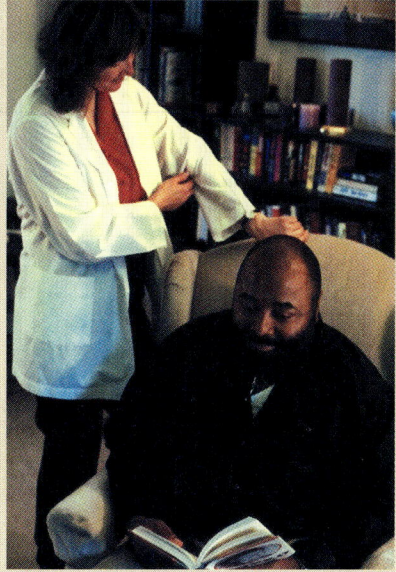

Figure 1-4-5 Count inspirations for a full 30 seconds.

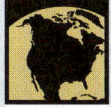

▶ **REAL WORLD ANECDOTES**

It is 6 AM and morning medication administration is well underway. The nurse caring for Carl enters the room to take his vital signs prior to giving him a dose of digoxin. Carl is still sleeping, and the nurse completes the pulse assessment without waking him. While attempting to count respirations she notes that Carl has stopped breathing. She feels for a pulse, which is still strong. After 45 seconds, Carl once again takes a breath. The nurse notes in Carl's chart that he appears to have sleep apnea. She leaves a note for Carl's physician regarding her observations and notes to herself the importance of counting respirations for at least 30 seconds.

▶ EVALUATION

- Evaluate client's respirations as a baseline value.
- Compare respirations with baseline to detect any alterations.

▶ DOCUMENTATION

Vital Signs Flow Sheet
- Respiratory rate

Nurses' Notes
- Record depth, rhythm, and character of respirations.
- Report a respiratory rate outside the normal age range, an irregular rhythm, inadequate depth, or any abnormal characteristics such as dyspnea.

▶ CRITICAL THINKING SKILL

Introduction
Assessing, but not correctly interpreting, abnormal respirations can lead to misdiagnosis or lack of treatment for a client.

Possible Scenario
While assessing clients at the beginning of the shift, the nursing student notes that Mr. Johnson, a diabetic, is lethargic. He responds to her greeting by asking where his baseball glove is. His respiration rate is 40 breaths per minute and his respirations are deep. His breath has a fruity odor. At the shift report, the nurse reported that he was alert and oriented with normal vital signs.

Possible Outcome
The student is glad that Mr. Johnson seems interested in his hobbies again, and seems to be so calm. She is reassured by his deep breathing, and is glad he was able to drink some apple juice. She leaves the room. Thirty minutes later, the respiratory therapist comes in and notes that Mr. Johnson is having Kussmaul's respirations and notifies Mr. Johnson's nurse. She instructs the student nurse to check Mr. Johnson's blood glucose level while she urgently notifies his physician of the serious deterioration in his condition. Failure to catch this change in Mr. Johnson's condition could have led to his death.

Prevention
Any vital signs outside normal limits need assessment and interpretation. The rapid change in this client's condition should further alert the nurse to trouble. Any significant or rapid change in a client's condition should be noted and reported immediately to the client's physician. In this case, the client was exhibiting Kussmaul's respirations (a marked increase in rate and depth of respiration), which is associated with severe diabetic acidosis.

▶ VARIATIONS

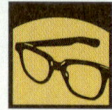

Geriatric Variations:
- *Geriatric clients may be confused, restless, or eager to talk so it may be difficult to get an opportunity to count quiet, at-rest respirations.*
- *Ask the client to sit quietly while you take his/her pulse or perhaps distract him/her with television or other activities.*

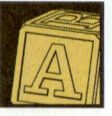

Pediatric Variations:
- *Counting respirations in small children should be done by observation.*
- *Give a small child a toy or something to distract him while you count his respirations.*
- *Infants or newborns at risk for respiratory arrest may need an apnea monitor at home.*

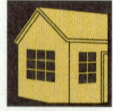

Home Care Variations:
- *Be sure the client is able to sit quietly while you take his vital signs to ensure an accurate reading.*
- *Assess the home for factors that may influence his breathing, such as ventilation or gas fumes.*

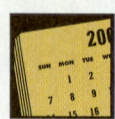

Long-Term-Care Variation:
- *Clients with long-term respiratory disease are often very aware of any changes to the air space around them. Do not stand in front of clients because it may cause them to feel as if you are cutting off their air supply, which could increase their respiratory rate and their anxiety.*

► COMMON ERRORS

Possible Error:
You take a resting respiration measurement of a client who is late for his appointment and who just walked up three flights of stairs instead of taking the elevator.

Prevention:
Be sure the client has at least 5–10 minutes to sit and rest to allow his vital signs to return to a resting state.

► NURSING TIPS

- Try not to stand directly in front of the client while counting respirations. Some clients feel as though it is harder to breathe when someone stands directly in front of them.
- Fear, pain, and anger can easily raise the respiratory rate. If these emotions are present, consider assessing the rate again at a later time when the client appears calmed.
- If possible, clients should not be aware you are counting their respirations, because such awareness may alter the respiratory rate. Placing your hand on the client's wrist gives the appearance of taking a pulse, and turns the client's attention away from your respiratory assessment.

► SPECIAL CONSIDERATIONS

- *Respirations are obtained in a variety of ways. The nurse might cross the client's hand across his/her chest as the pulse is obtained and then linger to count respirations. This is very helpful with shallow breathers or those whose respirations are not immediately visible.*
- *Be aware of the individual differences in breathing rate. Some clients such as athletes, might be trained to breath at a lower rate, e.g., at 6 breaths per minute. In respiration assessment, use the individual baseline and the established individual record for respiration evaluation.*

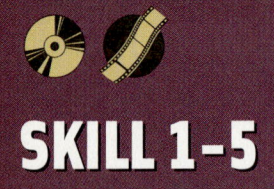

SKILL 1-5 Taking Blood Pressure

Karrin Johnson, RN, and Eileen M. Collins, RN, MN, ARNP

KEY TERMS

Auscultation	Korotkoff's sounds
Auscultatory gap	Palpation
Diastolic	Sphygmomanometer
Hypertension	Stethoscope
Hypotension	Systolic

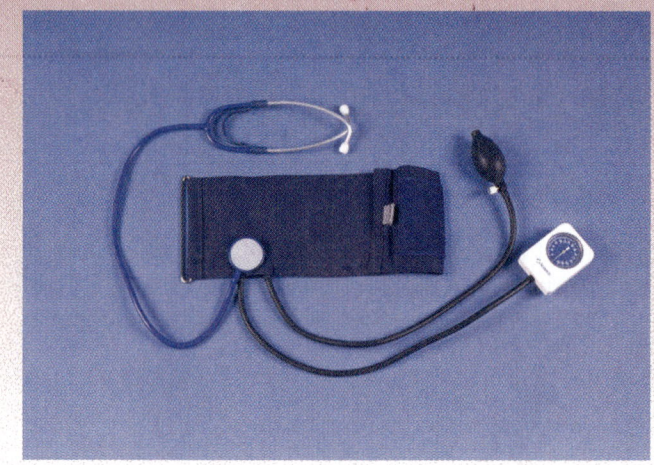

▸ OVERVIEW OF THE SKILL

Blood pressure measurement is performed during a physical examination, at initial assessment, and as part of routine vital signs assessment. Depending on the client's condition, the blood pressure is measured by either a direct or indirect technique.

The indirect method requires use of the sphygmomanometer and stethoscope for auscultation and palpation as needed. The most common site for indirect blood pressure measurement is the client's arm over the brachial artery. When the client's condition prevents auscultation of the brachial artery, the nurse should assess the blood pressure in the forearm or leg sites. When pressure measurements in the upper extremities are not accessible, the popliteal artery, located behind the knee, is the site of choice. The nurse can also assess blood pressure in other sites, such as the radial artery in the forearm and the posterior tibial or dorsalis pedis artery in the lower leg. Because it is difficult to auscultate sounds over the radial, tibial, and dorsalis pedis arteries, these sites are usually palpated to obtain a systolic reading.

The direct method requires an invasive procedure in which an intravenous catheter with an electronic sensor is inserted into an artery and the artery-transmitted pressure on an electronic display unit is read.

Hypotension is defined as a systolic blood pressure less than 90 mm Hg or 20 to 30 mm Hg below the adult client's normal systolic pressure. Orthostatic hypotension or postural hypotension refers to a sudden drop of 25 mm Hg in systolic pressure and a drop of 10 mm Hg in diastolic pressure when the client moves from a lying to a sitting position or from a sitting to a standing position.

Hypertension refers to a persistent systolic pressure greater than 135 to 140 mm Hg and a diastolic pressure greater than 90 mm Hg. For a diagnosis of hypertension to be made, the client must have a sustained elevation in blood pressure over a period of time.

▸ ASSESSMENT

1. Assess the condition of the potential blood pressure (BP) site **so that a site with an injury or surgery proximal to the site can be avoided.**
2. Assess the artery for any compromise to it **so that compressing the artery briefly will not cause decrease in circulation.**
3. Assess the distal pulse **to check if it is intact and palpable.**
4. Assess the circumference of the **extremity for the right size cuff to be used so an accurate reading can be obtained.**
5. Assess for factors that affect blood pressure, such as age, anxiety, fear, medications, smoking, eat-

SKILL 1-5 Taking Blood Pressure

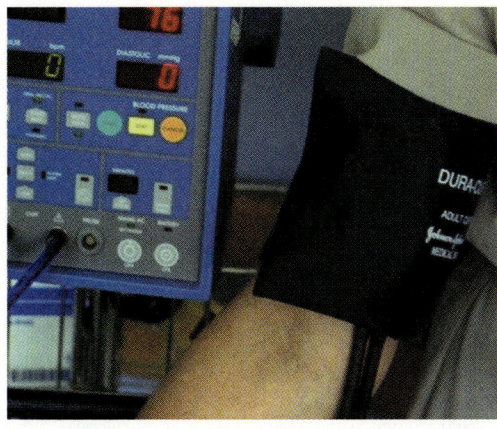

Figure 1-5-1 Be aware of blood pressure–related factors such as age, anxiety, and medications, prior to taking a blood pressure reading.

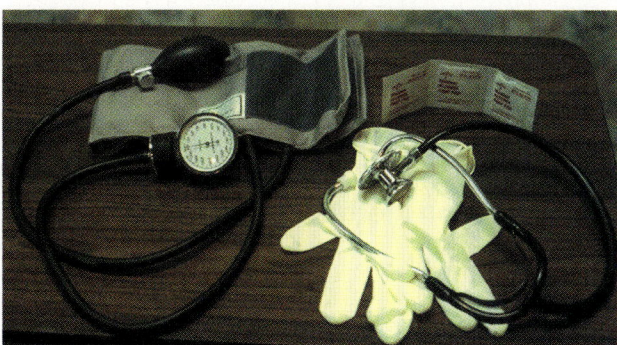

Figure 1-5-2 Sphygmomanometer, stethoscope, and gloves.

ing or exercising within 30 minutes prior to blood pressure assessment, and postural **changes so that an accurate reading can be obtained.**

6. Determine client's baseline blood pressure by reading the medical record **so that a comparison can be made with each blood pressure reading** (see Figure 1-5-1).

▶ DIAGNOSIS

- Ineffective Cardiopulmonary Tissue Perfusion.
- Decreased Cardiac Output.
- Knowledge Deficit of Blood Pressure Control.

▶ PLANNING

Expected Outcomes:

1. An accurate estimate of the arterial pressure at diastole and systole will be obtained.
2. Blood pressure is within normal range for the client.
3. Client will be able to understand why the blood pressure is taken and what it means.

Equipment Needed (see Figure 1-5-2):

- Stethoscope
- Sphygmanometer/bladder with mercury column or aneroid dial
- Gloves, if required
- Alcohol swabs

▶ CLIENT EDUCATION NEEDED

1. Teach the client to refrain from eating, drinking, or smoking 30 minutes before the procedure.
2. Ask the client to sit or lie down in a warm, quiet room.
3. Ask the client to rest for 5 minutes before taking the measurement.
4. Calmly explain the procedure.
5. Advise the client regarding the correct size blood pressure cuff to use at home for his/her individual anatomy.
6. Advise the client to take his/her blood pressure at the same site using the same cuff for consistency.
7. Teach the client that the "top number" in a blood pressure reading is always higher than the "bottom number."

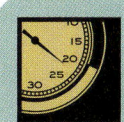 Estimated time to complete the skill: **5 minutes**

▶ DELEGATION TIPS

The measurement of blood pressure is often delegated to ancillary personnel who have been properly educated to use both manual and electronic equipment; however, the nurse is responsible for carefully monitoring this information for significant changes and taking appropriate action. The measurement of blood pressure would be reserved for a client in stable physical condition and measured at sites without intravenous solutions infusing, dialysis shunt or fistula, painful extremity, or recent mastectomy.

IMPLEMENTATION—ACTION/RATIONALE

ACTION	RATIONALE

Auscultation Method Using Brachial Artery

1. Wash hands.

2. Determine which extremity is most appropriate for reading. Do not take a pressure reading on an injured or painful extremity or one in which an intravenous line is running.

3. Select a cuff size appropriate for the client. Estimate by inspection, or measure with a tape, the circumference of the bare upper arm at the midpoint between the shoulder (acromium) and the elbow (olecranon process) (see Figure 1-5-3).

1. Reduces transmission of microorganisms.

2. Cuff inflation can temporarily interrupt blood flow and compromise circulation in an extremity already impaired or a vein receiving intravenous fluid.

3. The bladder inside the cuff should encircle 80% of the arm in adults and 100% of the arm of children less than 13 years old. If in doubt, use a larger cuff to ensure equalization of pressure on the artery and accurate measurement.

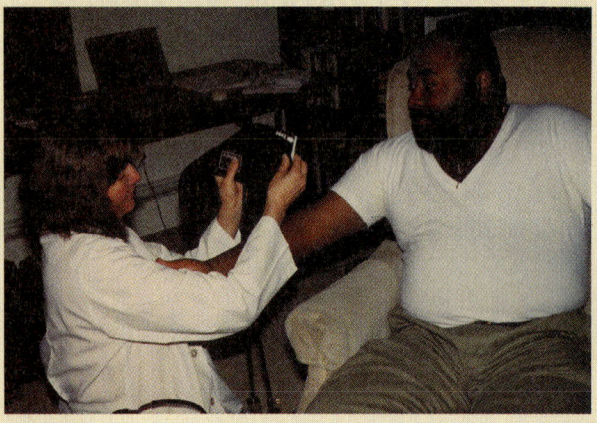

Figure 1-5-3 Select proper cuff size. An obese client may need a larger size cuff to obtain an accurate reading.

4. Have the client's bared arm resting on a support so the midpoint of the upper arm is at the level of the heart. Extend the elbow with palm turned upward.

5. Make sure the bladder cuff is fully deflated and the pump valve moves freely. Place the manometer so the center of the mercury column or aneroid dial is at eye level and easily visible to the observer.

6. Palpate the brachial artery, in the antecubital space, and place the cuff so that the midline of the bladder is over the arterial pulsation. Next, wrap and secure the cuff snugly around the client's bare upper arm. The lower edge of the cuff should be 1 inch (2 cm) above the antecu-

4. Blood pressure increases when the arm is below the level of the heart and decreases when the arm is above the level of the heart.

5. Equipment must be visible and function properly to obtain an accurate reading.

6. Ensures even pressure distribution over the brachial artery. Rolling up the sleeve may form a tourniquet around the upper arm. Always use a bare arm.

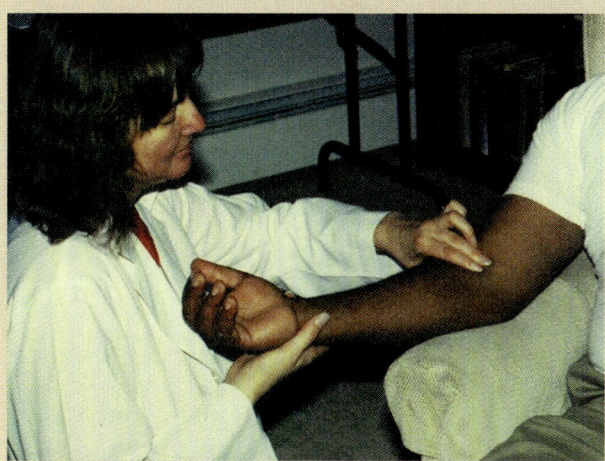

Figure 1-5-4 Palpate the brachial artery to determine placement of the stethoscope.

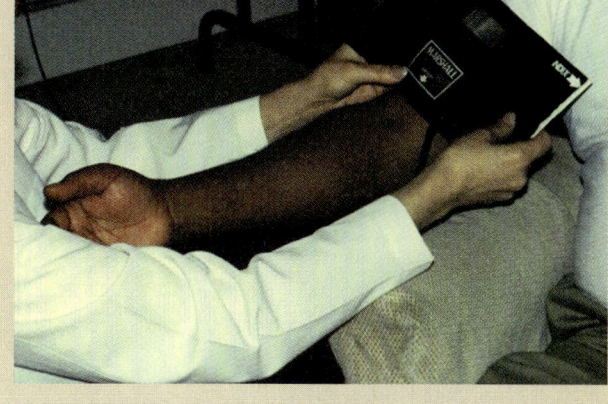

Figure 1-5-5 Center the blood pressure cuff over the brachial artery.

bital fossa (bend of the elbow), where the head of the stethoscope is to be placed (see Figures 1-5-4 and 1-5-5).

7. Inflate the cuff rapidly to 70 mm Hg and increase by 10-mm increments while palpating the radial pulse. Note the level of pressure at which the pulse disappears and subsequently reappears during deflation.

8. Insert the earpieces of the stethoscope into the ear canals with a forward tilt to fit snugly.

9. Relocate the brachial artery with your nondominant hand, and place the bell of the stethoscope over the brachial artery pulsation. The bell should be held firmly in place, ensuring that the head is in direct contact with the skin and not touching the cuff (see Figure 1-5-6).

7. The palpatory method provides the necessary preliminary approximation of systolic blood pressure to ensure an accurate reading. When frequent measurements are required, such as every 15 minutes, the palpatory method is generally not incorporated with each pressure check.

8. The bell, the low-frequency position of the stethoscope, enhances sound transmission from chest piece to ears.

9. Sound is heard best directly over the artery. Wedging the head of the stethoscope under

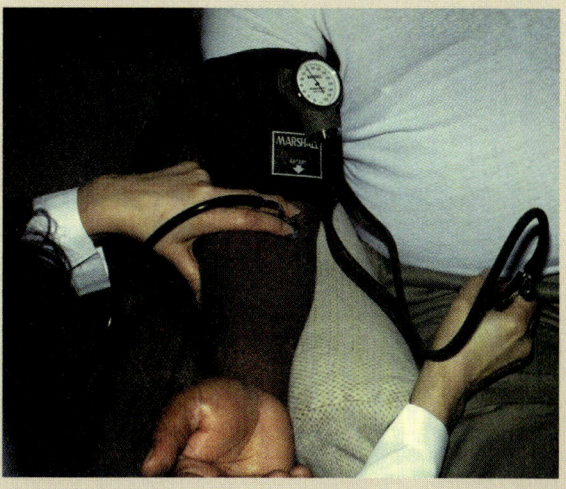

Figure 1-5-6 The stethoscope chestpiece should not touch the blood pressure cuff.

continues

Auscultation Method Using Brachial Artery
continued

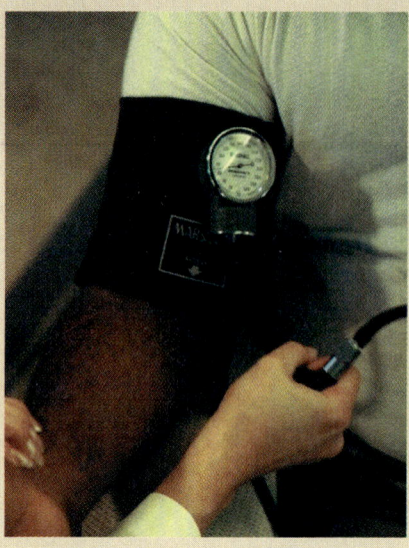

Figure 1-5-7 Compress the pump to inflate the blood pressure cuff.

10. With the dominant hand, turn the valve clockwise to close. Compress the pump to inflate the cuff rapidly and steadily until the manometer registers 20–30 mm Hg above the level previously determined by the palpation (see Figure 1-5-7).

11. Partially unscrew (open) the valve counterclockwise to deflate the bladder at 2 mm/sec while listening for the appearance of the five phases of the Korotkoff sounds. Note the manometer reading for these sounds.
    - I   A faint, clear tapping sound that increases in intensity can be heard.
    - II   Swishing sound.
    - III Intense sound.
    - IV   Abrupt, distinctive muffled sound.
    - V   Sound disappears.

(See Table 1-5-1 for more information about Korotkoff's sounds.)

12. After the last Korotkoff sound is heard, deflate the cuff slowly for at least another 10 mm Hg to ensure that no other sounds are audible; then, deflate rapidly and completely (see Figure 1-5-8).

the edge of the cuff results in considerable extraneous noise and may cause an inaccurate reading.

10. Prevents air leaks during inflation. Ensures the cuff is inflated to a pressure greater than the client's systolic pressure.

11. Maintains constant release of pressure to ensure hearing first systolic sound. Identify manometer readings for each of the five phases.
    - Identify two consecutive tapping sounds to confirm systolic reading.
    - The American Heart Association (2002) recommends using Phase IV as the diastolic level in children less than 13 years old. Even though 5 phases of Korotkoff sounds have been identified, most clients have only 2 clearly distinct sounds (phase I and V), identified as the systolic and diastolic sounds.

12. Prevents arterial occlusion and client discomfort from numbness or tingling.

SKILL 1-5 Taking Blood Pressure

Figure 1-5-8 Deflate the cuff completely and wait at least 2 minutes before taking a second reading.

13. Allow the client to rest for at least 30 seconds and remove cuff. (A measurement should be repeated after 30 seconds and the two readings averaged. It may be done in the same or opposite arm) (American Heart Association, 2002).

14. Inform the client of the reading.

15. The systolic (Phase I) and diastolic (Phase V) pressure should be immediately recorded, rounded off (upward) to the nearest 2 mm Hg. (In children and when sounds are heard nearly to the level of 0 mm Hg, the Phase IV pressure should also be recorded.)

16. If appropriate, lower bed, raise side rails, and place call light in easy reach.

17. Put all equipment in proper place.

18. Wash hands.

13. Releases trapped blood in the vessels. Ensures accurate measurement.

14. Promotes client's participation in health care.

15. Ensures accuracy.

16. Promotes client's safety.

17. Fosters maintenance of equipment.

18. Reduces transmission of microorganisms.

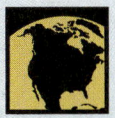

▶ REAL WORLD ANECDOTES

Scenario 1

While Mrs. Price's blood pressure is being taken, she complains of pain in her arm. When Mrs. Price is questioned regarding the pain, she reports that about 5 years earlier she broke her shoulder and her arm has been sensitive ever since. When asked why she had not communicated this to the nurse prior to the blood pressure reading, Mrs. Price indicated that she assumed the nurse knew best. Be aware of individual client variations, especially when performing routine tasks.

continues

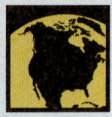

> ► **REAL WORLD ANECDOTES** continued
>
> **Scenario 2**
>
> *Mr. Johnson came to the occupational health nurse at his company to have his blood pressure checked as part of a company-wide campaign. His reading was very high. Upon further discussion, he told the nurse that he had just had a very frustrating argument over some purchase orders with a customer at lunch. He was stuck in traffic and had to run in from the parking lot to make this appointment. The nurse asked him to sit quietly for a few minutes, then took his blood pressure a second time. It was much lower, and within normal limits. Clients who have recently eaten, ambulated, or experienced an emotional upset will have a falsely high blood pressure reading.*

► EVALUATION

- Evaluate the blood pressure reading for accuracy by comparing with the medical record.
- Evaluate the client's blood pressure for being within the normal range.
- Identify variations in the client's blood pressure of more than 5 to 10 mm Hg from one arm to the other.
- Evaluate if the client's blood pressure changes significantly when he/she stands up.
- Report abnormal measurements to charge nurse, physician, or qualified practitioner.

► DOCUMENTATION

Vital Signs Flow Sheet

- Record the blood pressure measurement.
- Record the site where recording was done.
- Record the method of obtaining the pressure—auscultation or palpation.

► CRITICAL THINKING SKILL

Introduction

The routine of taking a blood pressure may become a mindless task. It is an important physical assessment tool.

Possible Scenario

Paul is a morbidly obese middle-aged client. He has a history of Type II diabetes and hypertension. He is being admitted to the hospital for observation of his blood sugar and blood pressure. You are performing his admission evaluation including vital signs. You use a blood pressure cuff that is in the room to take Paul's blood pressure, even though it barely covers his arm.

Possible Outcome

Your reading shows a drastically elevated blood pressure—the admitting orders call for transfer to intensive care and Nipride therapy for a blood pressure this high. The client reports that when he took his pressure earlier in the day it was much lower. You ask another nurse to check Paul's blood pressure. He notes that the cuff you used is too small for Paul's arm and brings the correct size cuff from the nurses' station. This reading is much lower. Subsequent readings with the correct-sized cuff show no immediate intervention is necessary.

Prevention

A blood pressure reading must be accurate to be an effective diagnostic tool. Taking a blood pressure reading on obese patients with an average-sized adult cuff can give a falsely elevated reading. In addition, a blood pressure cuff that is too small for the client's arm will often come unfastened as it is inflated. Be sure to use the correct-sized cuff for the client.

► VARIATIONS

Geriatric Variations:

- *The systolic blood pressure may be overestimated by the indirect method of measurement due to sclerotic, calcified vessels. If the brachial artery is readily palpable, even when the cuff is inflated and the blood flow is interrupted (positive Olser's sign), then the measurement may not be accurate. Under these circumstances an incorrect diagnosis of hypertension may be made. Direct measurement should be used for confirmation.*

▶ VARIATIONS continued

- Postural hypotension is often observed in the elderly.
- Elderly clients may have lost muscle mass, and their upper arms may be quite thin. Be sure to adjust the cuff size to accommodate the client's arm.
- Many elderly clients have a history of hypertension and are taking antihypertensive medications.

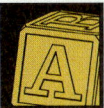

Pediatric Variations:
- Determine the diastolic pressure as Phase IV in children under 13 years of age, because the Korotkoff sounds are often heard through the entire period of deflation.
- The palpatory method is often used for approximating systolic pressure in small children and infants; however, the measurement may be 5 to 10 mm Hg lower than the level measured by auscultation.
- Small children may be uncooperative with the procedure and need the assistance of a parent/adult to hold still.
- A cuff that fits adequately may not be available to ensure that the bladder completely encircles the limb. It may be preferable to use the popliteal artery when taking a child's blood pressure.
- Blood pressure varies with size as the child reaches adolescence.
- Take a blood pressure first before anxiety- or pain-producing procedures.

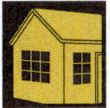

Home Care Variations:
- Use the same blood pressure cuff the client normally uses for home readings.
- Compare the client's home readings to a reading obtained with a cuff that you know is properly calibrated.
- Assess the client's financial ability to buy his/her own sphygmomanometer.
- Consider use of an electric blood pressure cuff if the client has a hearing deficit.

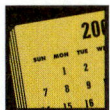

Long-Term-Care Variation:
- Be aware of any injuries, disease processes, or medical devices (such as stents) that may contraindicate a blood pressure reading at the chosen site.

▶ COMMON ERRORS

Possible Error:
When taking a blood pressure reading the cuff is low enough on the arm that the stethoscope bell must be slid underneath the bottom edge of the cuff to be properly placed over the artery.

Prevention:
Make sure to use the correct-sized cuff and that it is positioned correctly on the client to prevent the stethoscope from contacting the cuff. If you find that it is incorrectly applied, remove the cuff, assess cuff size, and reapply the correct-sized cuff, fitting it firmly on the upper arm so that the antecubital space is visible. Repeat the blood pressure reading.

▶ NURSING TIPS

- Do not take an blood pressure on an arm with an arteriovenous shunt, IV, or if the client has a history of surgery or injury to the breast, axilla, or arm.
- The tubes extending from the blood pressure cuff bladder are not always centered on the bladder itself. It is not accurate to assume that the area between these tubes represents the center of the cuff

- bladder. Be sure to center the bladder by palpating the bladder itself.
- False high readings occur when the mercury column in the manometer is not positioned flat on a firm surface, when it is read above eye level, or when the extremity is below the heart's apex level.
- False low readings occur when the extremity is above the heart's apex level, when the cuff is too wide for the extremity, or when the mercury column in the manometer is read below eye level.
- If the nurse fails to recognize the auscultatory gap, the temporary disappearance of sounds at the end of Korotkoff's Phase I and beginning of Phase II, the systolic pressure is read at a false low.
- There are many different types and brands of blood pressure measurement devices. Become familiar with the ones you will be working with.
- If an electronic blood pressure device is used, be sure to assess the accuracy of the machine. Use the same equipment when comparing a client's blood pressure.

▶ **SPECIAL CONSIDERATIONS**

- *Pulsus paradoxus*, also called paradoxic pulse, is an abnormal decrease (more than 10 mm Hg) in the systolic pressure and a decrease in pulse wave amplitude during inspiration. An excessive decline may be a sign of tamponade, adhesive pericarditis, severe lung disease, heart failure, or other conditions.
- Ask the client what his/her normal blood pressure is, and use it not only as a gauge for cuff inflation but as an opportunity to teach the client about healthy blood pressure values.
- A child's blood pressure may vary with age. A very low diastolic pressure is not always indicative of underlying cardiac disease.
- An alternative method when taking a blood pressure in a very small infant, when Doppler or automated oscillometric equipment is unavailable, is the flush method. The American Heart Association (2002) defines this as follows: "placing a suitable cuff on the arm or leg, raising the limb, and wrapping the extremity distal to the cuff firmly with an elastic bandage until it is drained of blood and blanches. The limb is then lowered to heart level, the cuff is rapidly inflated, and the bandage is removed. As the pressure in the cuff is gradually reduced, flushing of the limb indicates the level at which the flow returns. This level corresponds to mean blood pressure but is inaccurate in infants with anemia, hypothermia, or edema."
- Blood pressure should be taken in the alternate arm in clients who have recently had a mastectomy with extensive axillary node dissection or other surgical procedure involving the arm or shoulder. In dialysis patients, the alternate arm should be used when the client has an arteriovenous fistula.

Table 1-5-1 Korotkoff's Sounds Correlated to Pressure Dynamics

PHASE	PRESSURE DYNAMICS
I: Clear, soft tapping that increases to a thud or loud tap (systolic sound).	Ventilation—the inflow and outflow of air between the atmosphere and the lung alveoli.
II: Tapping changes to a soft, swishing sound.	Circulation—the quantity of blood flowing through the lungs equals that flowing through systemic circulation.
III: Clear tapping sound returns.	Diffusion—the exchange of oxygen and carbon dioxide between the alveoli and the blood.
IV: Muffled, blowing sound (diastolic sound in children or physically active adults).	Transport—the carrying of oxygen and carbon dioxide in the blood and body fluids to and from the cells.
V: Disappearance of muffled, blowing sound (second diastolic sound).	Regulation—the neurogenic system that adjusts the rate of alveolar ventilation to meet the demands of the body.

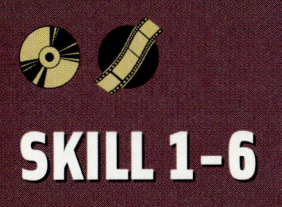

SKILL 1-6

Weighing a Client, Mobile and Immobile

Bethany Campbell, RN, MN and Gaylene Bouska Altman, RN, PhD

KEY TERMS

Calibrate
Sling scale
Standing balance scale
Standing electronic scale
Weight

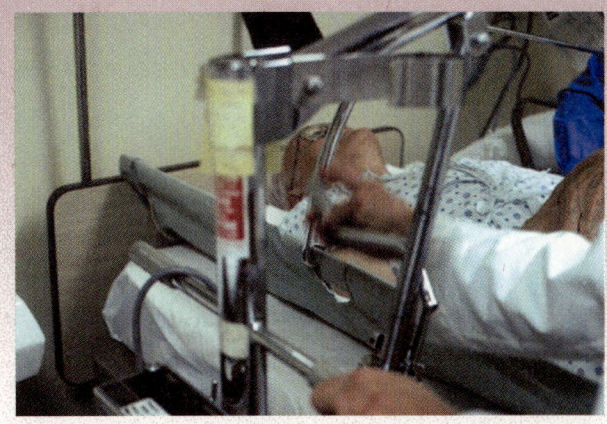

▶ OVERVIEW OF THE SKILL

A client's weight is an essential piece of data used in monitoring his response to a variety of therapies. Changes in a client's weight could necessitate an alteration in the assessment and intervention plans. An accurate weight is important, therefore, to ensure appropriate care.

▶ ASSESSMENT

1. Assess the client's ability to stand independently and safely on a scale. **Consider factors requiring the use of a sling scale: the client is somnolent or comatose; paralyzed; too weak to stand; or unsteady when standing.**
2. Determine if clothing is similar to that worn during previous weight measurement **to help determine accuracy of the new weight.**

▶ DIAGNOSIS

- Imbalanced Nutrition: More than Body Requirements.
- Imbalanced Nutrition: Less than Body Requirements.
- Excess Fluid Volume.
- Deficient Fluid Volume

▶ PLANNING

Expected Outcomes:

1. Health care provider obtains accurate weight.
2. Client incurs no injuries.
3. Client maintains privacy.

Equipment Needed:

- Scale: standing electronic or balance scale (see Figure 1-6-1); or sling scale (see Figure 1-6-2)
- Recommended disinfectant
- 1–3 other staff members to assist when using sling scale
- Plastic cover for sling scale
- Gloves (when applicable)

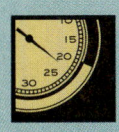 Estimated time to complete the skill:
3 minutes when using standing scale
10 minutes when using sling scale

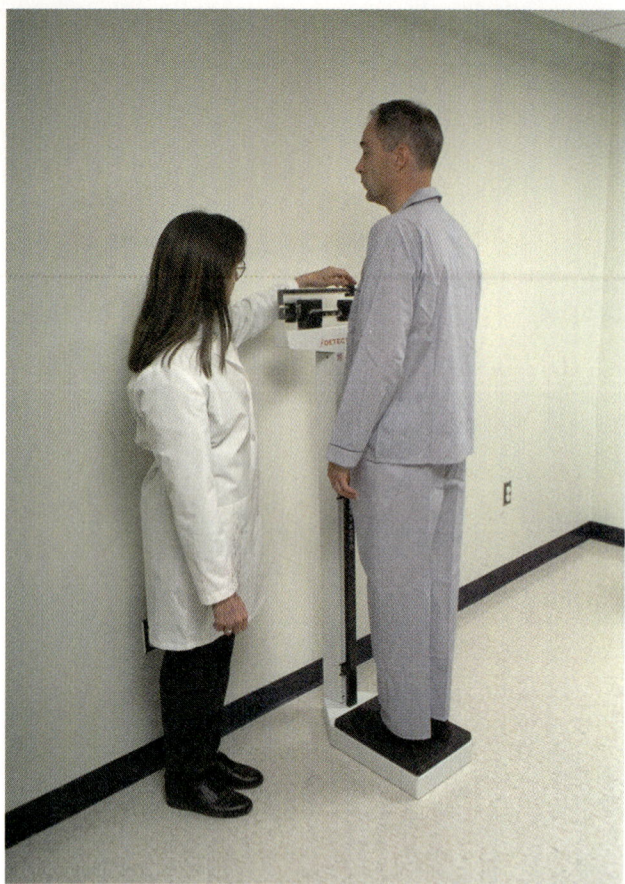

Figure 1-6-1 The standing balance scale is used to weigh ambulatory clients.

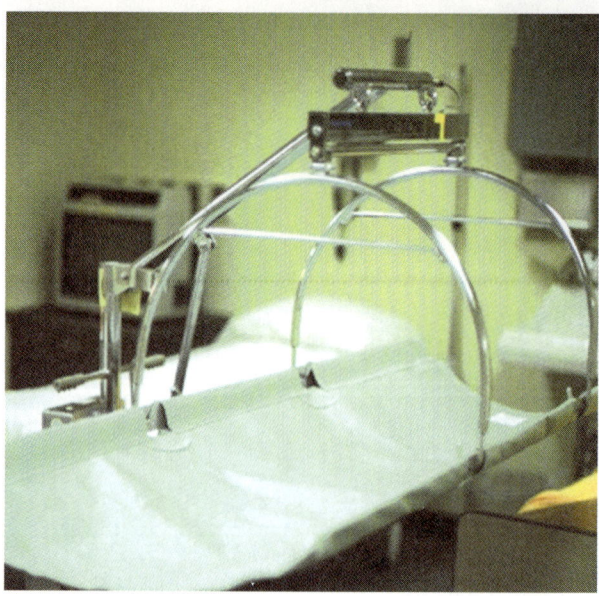

Figure 1-6-2 The sling scale is used to weigh clients in bed.

▶ CLIENT EDUCATION NEEDED

1. When using the standing electronic scale, instruct the client not to step onto the scale until the digital display reads zero.
2. When using the sling scale, incorporate clients as you go through the procedure. Provide instructions when asking clients to turn, and be sure to inform clients before lifting.
3. Instruct clients in the correct way to monitor weight at home, i.e., by weighing themselves without clothes first thing in the morning after voiding.
4. Remind clients weighing themselves at home to use the scales on the same, even hard surface (kitchen or bathroom tile, hardwood floor).

▶ DELEGATION TIPS

The skill of weighing the mobile and immobile client is routinely delegated to trained ancillary personnel. The personnel should be instructed to do the following:
- Select the correct scale for measurement.
- Properly and safely position the client for measurement.
- Correctly and safely perform the measurement according to established guidelines and record on the appropriate flow sheet (clinical record).
- Recognize and report abnormal findings promptly to the nurse.

SKILL 1-6 Weighing a Client, Mobile and Immobile

IMPLEMENTATION—ACTION/RATIONALE

ACTION	RATIONALE
Standing Scale	
1. Wash hands.	1. Reduces transmission of microorganisms.
2. Introduce yourself to the client and explain what you would like him/her to do.	2. Builds rapport; involves the client in care.
3. Place the scale near the client.	3. Reduces risk of fall or injury.
4. Turn on the scale, and calibrate it to zero.	4. Ensures accurate reading.
5. Ask client to remove shoes if necessary step up on the scale, and stand still (see Figure 1-6-3). *Electronic scale:* Read weight after digital numbers have stopped fluctuating. *Balance scale:* Slide the larger weight into the notch most closely approximating the client's weight. Slide the smaller weight into the notch such that the balance rests in the middle. Add the two numbers to read the client's weight.	5. Obtains weight. Reading is not accurate when the numbers are still fluctuating. Weights on scale must be balanced to obtain accurate reading.
6. Ask the client to step down. Assist the client back to the bed or chair, if necessary.	6. Reduces risk of injury if client needs assistance.
7. Wipe the scale with appropriate disinfectant.	7. Reduces risk of spread of infection.
8. Wash hands.	8. Reduces transmission of microorganisms.

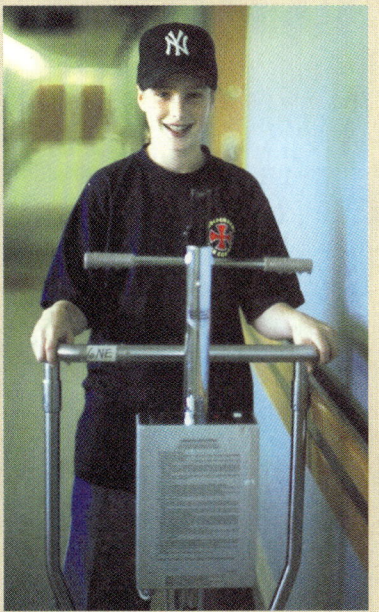

Figure 1-6-3 Have client stand straight and still while on the standing scale to obtain accurate measurements of weight and height.

continues

Sling Scale

9. Wash hands and put on gloves if appropriate.

9. Reduces risk of nosocomial infection.

10. Introduce yourself to the client and explain what you would like /her to do.

10. Builds rapport; involves the client in care.

11. Place plastic covering on sling if available (can usually be ordered in bulk from the manufacturer).

11. Reduces risk of spreading infection between clients.

12. Remove pillows. Turn the client to one side and place half of sling on bed next to the client, with remaining half rolled up against the client's back (see Figure 1-6-4).

12. Most accurate weight will be obtained by leaving no other bedding between the client and sling.

13. Turn the client to the other side, and unroll the rest of the sling so it lays flat beneath the client.

13. Turning in this manner maximizes client comfort.

14. Roll the scale over the bed such that the legs of the scale are underneath the bed (see Figure 1-6-5). Open and lock the legs of the scale.

14. Ensures equipment is being used safely to reduce risk of injury.

15. Turn on scale and calibrate to zero.

15. Ensures accurate reading.

16. Lower arms of the scale and slip hooks through holes in sling (see Figure 1-6-6).

16. Attaches sling to scale to obtain weight.

17. Pump scale until sling rests completely off the bed (see Figure 1-6-7).

17. Ensures accurate weight.

18. Remind the client to remain still. Read weight after digital numbers have stopped fluctuating (see Figure 1-6-8).

18. Reading is not accurate when the numbers are still fluctuating.

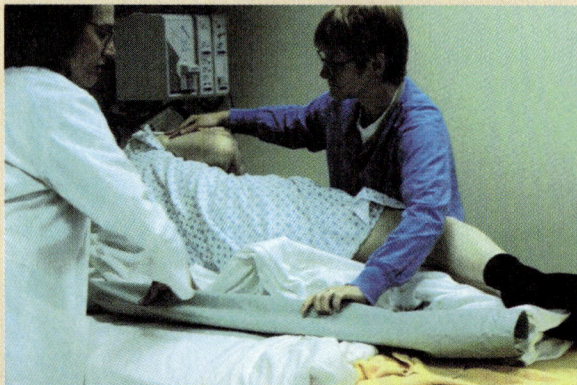

Figure 1-6-4 Turn client on one side, and place sling on the bed.

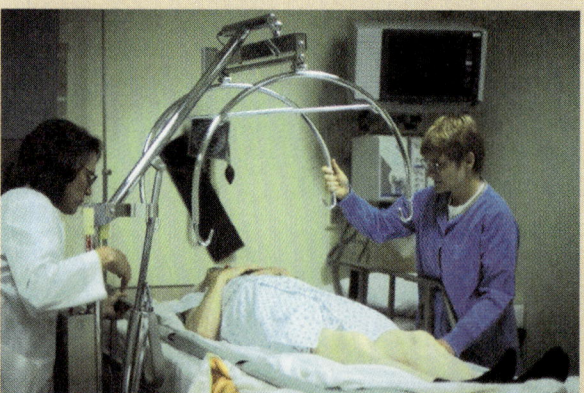

Figure 1-6-5 After unrolling the rest of the sling under the client, move the scale into position over the bed.

SKILL 1-6 Weighing a Client, Mobile and Immobile

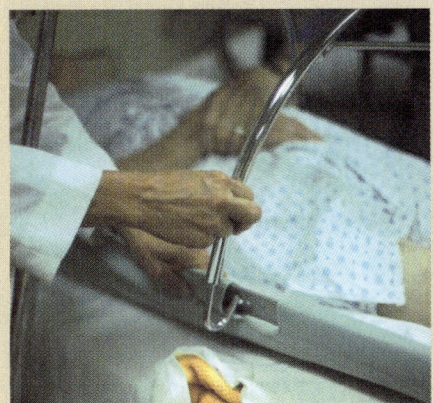

Figure 1-6-6 Attach the hooks through the holes in the sling.

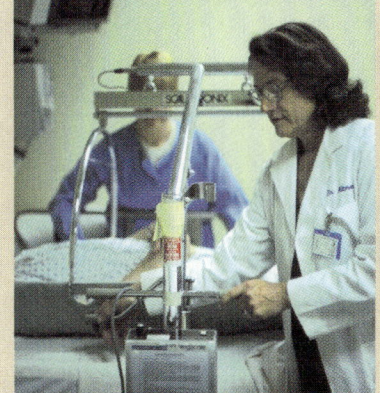

Figure 1-6-7 Pump the scale until the sling lifts completely off the bed.

19. Lower the client back to bed, and remove arms of the scale from sling (see Figure 1-6-9).

20. Unlock legs, return to their original position, and remove scale from bed.

21. Turn the client on his/her side, roll up sling, turn client to the other side.

22. Realign the client with pillows and covers.

23. Remove plastic covering from the sling and discard as per hospital policy.

24. Remove gloves and wash hands.

25. Wash hands.

19. Prepare for removal of sling.

20. Allows for removal of equipment that obstructs proximity to the client, thereby facilitating removal of the sling.

21. Facilitates removal of the sling.

22. Ensures comfort and privacy.

23. Reduces risk of spread of infection.

24. Reduces risk of nosocomial infection.

25. Reduces transmission of microorganisms.

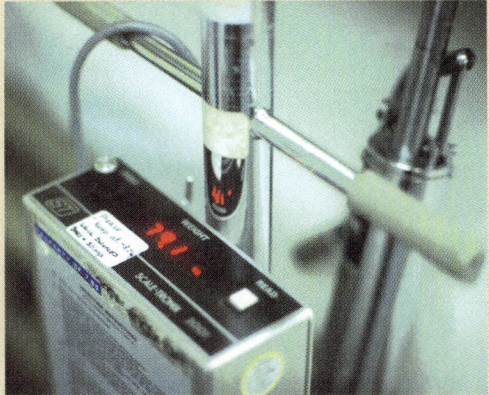

Figure 1-6-8 Read the weight after the numbers have stopped fluctuating.

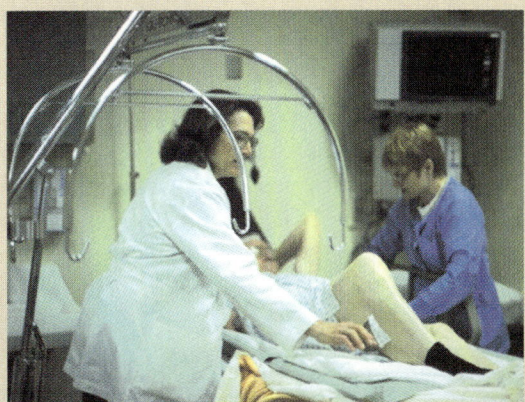

Figure 1-6-9 Lower the client back to the bed, and remove the sling.

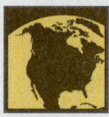

> ► **REAL WORLD ANECDOTES**
> A client was called back to the exam room area. The nurse wanted to check her weight on the standing scale in the hallway. The client was very upset that the nurse wanted to weigh her with her shoes on, which would add pounds to her weight. The nurse needed to hear that this individual was concerned and embarrassed about being overweight.

► EVALUATION

- Compare weight obtained to previously recorded weight. Repeat weight if large discrepancy noted.
- If large discrepancy still remains, notify appropriate health care team members.

► DOCUMENTATION

Vital Signs Flow Sheet

- Record the date, time of day, and the weight of the client on the appropriate flow sheet.

► CRITICAL THINKING SKILL

Introduction

Dramatic weight fluctuation may be explored by improper technique.

Possible Scenario

An immobile client has just been weighed using an over-the-bed scale. The nurse is alarmed that the client seems to have lost 20 pounds in 2 days. She records her findings in the nurses' notes and alerts the nurse practitioner.

Possible Outcome

The nurse practitioner comes and repeats the weight. She finds the client has actually gained a pound. Upon reviewing her technique, the nurse realizes that she probably did not lift the scale sling high enough to clear the bed, resulting in an inaccurate weight.

Prevention

Lift the sling high enough so that no part of the client touches the bed. Double-check any large change in weight with no apparent cause.

► VARIATIONS

Geriatric Variation:
- *Elderly clients may need more assistance when moving to the scale. Consider using a sling scale if the client is too unsteady to stand independently.*

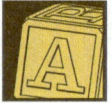

Pediatric Variation:
- *Pediatric scales are necessary to weigh infants. Follow the same steps as for a standing electronic scale, except place the infant on the scale after ensuring calibration, and elicit the caregiver's assistance in calming and distracting the child.*

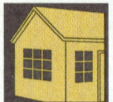

Home Care Variations:
- *When using a client's own scale, assess its proper functioning, and use it in a consistent manner to ensure accuracy. For example, weigh the client using the scale on the same hard, even surface for each reading (e.g., bathroom or kitchen tile, hardwood floor).*
- *If you bring your own scale to a home visit, compare the two scales prior to recording weights from the different scales on the same flow sheet.*
- *Home scales may need to be adjusted so they read "0" when there is no weight on the scale.*

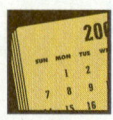

Long-Term-Care Variations:
- *Establish an appropriate weigh schedule for the long-term-care client. It is easy to forget to weigh a client. Keeping an accurate weight will help monitor long-term gains or losses.*
- *Keeping a current weight will establish a baseline to compare with future changes.*

▶ COMMON ERRORS

Possible Errors:

Weight obtained differs greatly from previously recorded weight.

Prevention:

Be sure the scale is appropriately calibrated prior to use. Recalibrate the scale and repeat the weight.

Possible Errors:

Sling scale begins to tip when the client is lifted off the bed.

Prevention:

Be sure to open the legs of the scale to broaden its support base. Lower the client, check scale legs, and open them if necessary.

▶ NURSING TIPS

- Weigh clients at the same time each day to enhance accuracy.
- Weigh clients in similar clothing each time to avoid unnecessary discrepancies.
- In an unfamiliar setting, check the bed. Some have a built-in scale.
- If a battery-operated electronic scale is used, plug it in between uses to keep the battery charged.

▶ SPECIAL CONSIDERATIONS

- *If the situation permits, use the same scale each time to ensure the measurement validity.*
- *When using the sling scale it is important to assess the environment, because as the hooks that slide through the holes can easily catch on surrounding objects.*
- *Be aware of added lines, dressings, and bedding when trying to gauge an accurate weight.*
- *Many types of scales are on the market. Check directions for accurate use and calibration.*

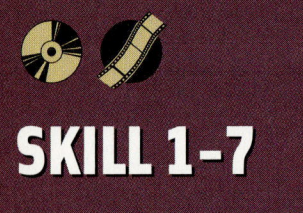

SKILL 1-7

Measuring Intake and Output

Karrin Johnson, RN and Gaylene Bouska Altman, RN, PhD

KEY TERMS

Dehydration
Fluid balance
Fluid retention
Intake
Output

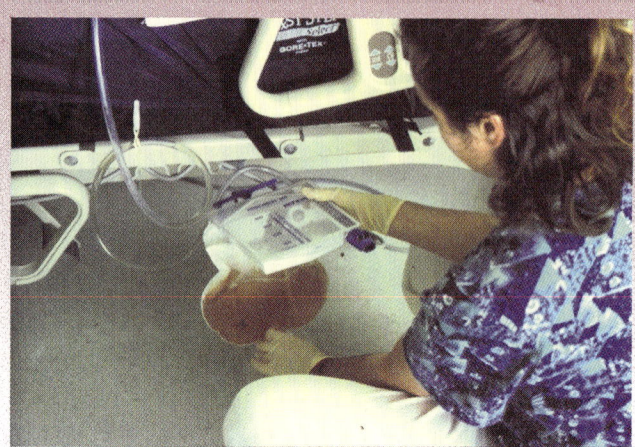

▶ OVERVIEW OF THE SKILL

One of the most basic methods of monitoring a client's health is measuring intake and output, commonly called "I and O." By monitoring the amount of fluids a client takes in and comparing this to the amount of fluid a client puts out, the health care team can gain valuable insights into the client's general health as well as monitor specific disease conditions.

To maintain good health, fluid intake should approximately equal fluid output. Intake that exceeds output can indicate medical conditions ranging from renal failure to congestive heart failure. Output that exceeds intake can be caused by things as serious as life-threatening diarrhea or as benign as diuretic medications. An accurate record of a client's fluid balance is an important nursing function.

Intake and output monitoring is often ordered by the physician or qualified practitioner but can also be initiated by the nurse. Some institutions have policies regarding conditions that require intake and output monitoring as well. Generally clients who are receiving fluids through any route other than oral or who are losing fluids through any route other than voiding are placed on intake and output measurement. Clients with conditions that affect fluid balance—i.e., diabetes, renal failure, diuretic therapy, or anorexia—also require intake and output monitoring.

Ideally intake and output should be monitored over several days to obtain an accurate record of the client's status. In critical situations, however, this may not be possible and the patient's intake and output may be monitored and reported on an hourly basis. A urine output of less than 30 cc per hour should be reported.

Daily weights are often done in conjunction with intake and output. Daily weights can indicate fluid retention or loss. One gallon of water weighs 8 pounds. An 8-pound weight gain over a 24–48-hour period could indicate a life-threatening condition for the client. A significant change in a client's weight or a significant difference in a client's total intake and output should be reported to the patient's physician or qualified practitioner.

Intake is considered to be any fluid consumed or infused. This includes water, juice, coffee, milk, ice cream, soup broth, and Jell-O®. Be sure to calculate the amount of water the client has consumed from the bedside water pitcher. Any fluids infused through IV lines, central lines, feeding tubes, or irrigant that is not returned is considered intake. Blood and blood products as well as the saline used to flush IV lines before and after the transfusion are also included in this count. IV piggybacks, fluids used to measure cardiac output, central line flushes, and *TKO* (to keep open) fluids are also considered in the intake total.

Urine is the largest component of output fluid volume, but there are a number of other fluid loss avenues that must be considered. Diarrhea, diaphoresis, wound drainage, gastric or other fluids removed by suction, and bleeding are all fluid losses as well. These losses should be measured or estimated and recorded in the total output.

Clients who are able to understand and cooperate with the intake and output measurement, should be encouraged to keep track of their fluid balance. Particularly in clients who are on a fluid restriction, client understanding and participation can greatly increase cooperation.

▶ ASSESSMENT

1. Assess the client's risk factors for fluid overload, such as congestive heart failure, renal failure, or ascites **because edema can result from excess volume in extracellular fluid spaces and transferring of fluid into tissues.**
2. Determine if the client is receiving fluids or medications that would predispose him to fluid overload such as large amounts of IV fluids or steroid therapy **because steroids cause sodium and water retention and excretion of potassium.**
3. Assess the client's risk factors for fluid loss such as diaphoresis, rapid respirations, diarrhea, gastric suction, blood loss, or wound drainage **because dehydration can result from reduction of fluid within the tissues and circulatory system.**
4. Determine if the client's urine output is in excess of his fluid intake **because the kidneys excrete excess fluid during periods of overhydration and conserve body water during periods of dehydration.**
5. Assess the client's ability to understand and cooperate with intake and output measurement **because cooperation in these measurements will help ensure accuracy.**

▶ DIAGNOSIS

- Excess Fluid Volume.
- Deficient Fluid Volume.
- Risk for Deficient Fluid Volume.

▶ PLANNING

Expected Outcomes:

1. The client's fluid intake and output will be accurately measured and recorded.
2. The client will participate in the recording of fluid intake and output if possible.

Equipment Needed (see Figure 1-7-1):

- I&O form at bedside
- I&O graphic record in chart
- Glass or cup
- Bedpan or urinal bedside commode
- Graduated container for output
- Nonsterile gloves
- Sign at bedside stating patient is on I&O

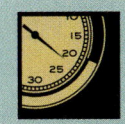 Estimated time to complete the skill: **5–10 minutes.**

▶ CLIENT EDUCATION NEEDED

1. Instruct the client how to measure fluid intake using standardized volumes of glassware and dishes.
2. Teach the client which intake is considered to be fluid and which is not. Remind the client what is considered fluid intake, e.g., coffee, tea, and soda pop, as well as gelatin, ice cream, and Popsicles.
3. Teach the client to measure and record the amount of fluid his standard utensils hold and then to use those utensils exclusively.
4. Instruct the client to void into a bedpan or urinal, not into a toilet.
5. Teach the client to dispose of toilet tissue in a plastic-lined container, not in the bedpan.

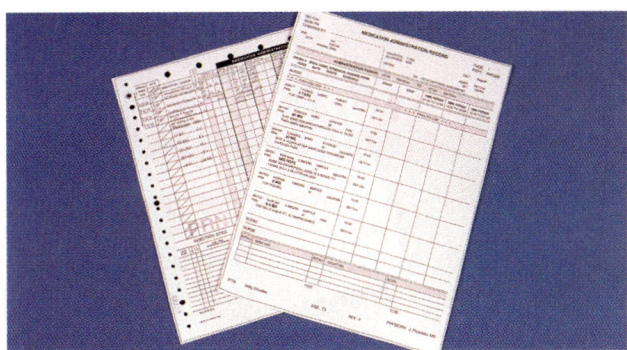

Figure 1-7-1 Intake and output forms.

▶ DELEGATION TIPS

Intake and output measurement may be delegated to ancillary personnel who should be knowledgable regarding the following:
- *Obtaining accurate measurements and reporting incontinence.*
- *Observing the amount, color, and any odor from the output.*
- *Protecting themselves from contamination from a body fluid and storing collection containers in designated areas.*
- *Recording measurements on proper clinical records.*

IMPLEMENTATION—ACTION/RATIONALE

ACTION	RATIONALE
1. Wash hands.	1. Reduces transmission of microorganisms.
2. Explain the rules of I&O record. All fluids taken orally must be recorded on the client's intake and output form (sometimes called a fluid balance flow sheet). • Client must void into bedpan or urinal, not into toilet (see Figures 1-7-2 and 1-7-3). • Toilet tissue should be disposed of in plastic-lined container, not in bedpan.	2. Elicits patient support. • Fluid voided into the toilet cannot be measured. • Liquids absorbed into toilet tissue cannot be measured by volume.

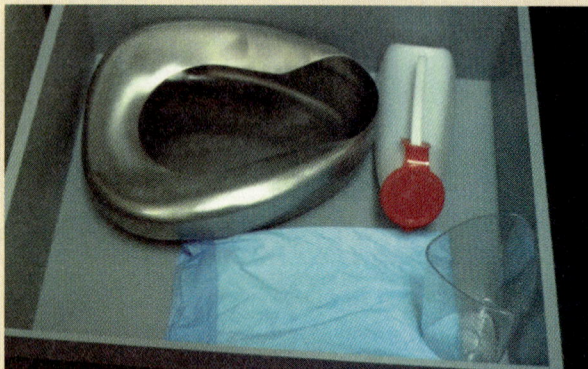

Figure 1-7-2 Bedpan and urinal, protective pad, and graduated specimen container.

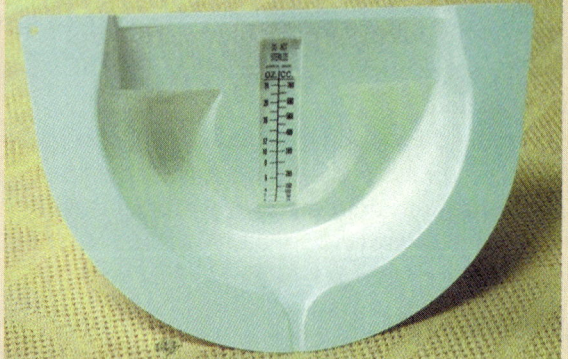

Figure 1-7-3 Graduated specimen container is used to measure urine, drainage, or other output.

3. Measure all oral fluids in accord with agency policy; e.g., cup = 150 ml, glass = 240 ml. Record all IV fluids as they are infused (see Figure 1-7-4).	3. Provides for consistency of measurement.
4. Record time and amount of all fluid intake in the designated space on bedside form (oral, tube feedings, IV fluids).	4. Documents fluids.

SKILL 1-7 Measuring Intake and Output

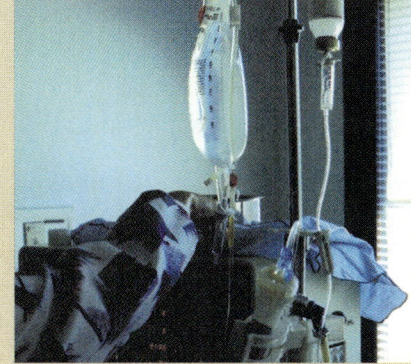

Figure 1-7-4 All IV infused fluids must be measured.

5. Transfer 8-hour total fluid intake from bedside I&O record to graphic sheet or 24-hour I&O record on client's chart.	5. Provides for data analysis of the client's fluid status.
6. Record all fluid intake, in the appropriate column of the 24-hour record.	6. Documents intake by type and amount.
7. Complete 24-hour intake record by adding all 8-hour totals.	7. Provides consistent data for analysis of the client's fluid status over a 24-hour period.

Output

8. Apply nonsterile gloves.	8. Reduces potential for transmission of pathogens.
9. Empty urinal, bedpan, or Foley drainage bag (see Figure 1-7-5) into graduated container or commode "hat" (see Figure 1-7-6).	9. Provides accurate measurement of urine.

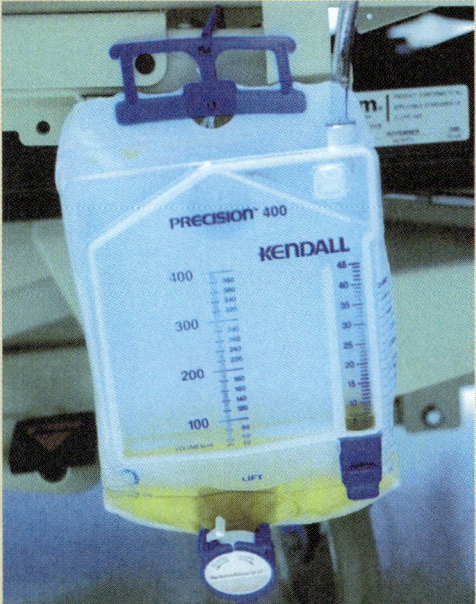

Figure 1-7-5 Urine in Foley drainage bag must be measured.

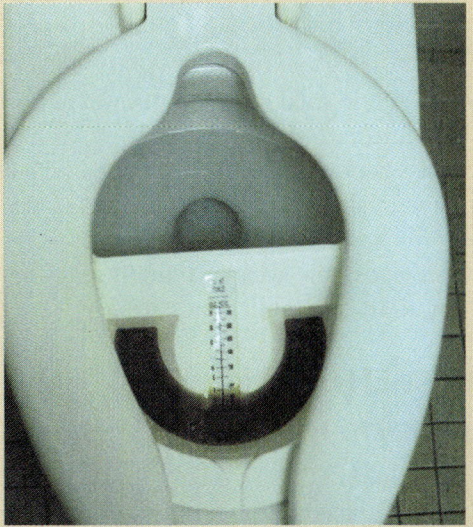

Figure 1-7-6 Empty urine into a graduated container to measure.

continues

Output *continued*

10. Remove gloves, and wash hands.	10. Prevents cross-contamination.
11. Record time and amount of output (urine, drainage from nasogastric tube, drainage tube) on I&O record.	11. Documents output.
12. Transfer 8-hour output totals to graphic sheet or 24-hour I&O record on the client's chart.	12. Provides for data analysis of the client's fluid status.
13. Complete 24-hour output record by totaling all 8-hour totals.	13. Provides consistent data for analysis of the client's fluid status over a 24-hour period.
14. Wash hands.	14. Reduces transmission of microorganisms.

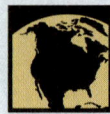

▶ **REAL WORLD ANECDOTES**

Mr. Aguilar is a critically ill patient in the coronary care unit. During the night his nurse noted that his urinary output was 10 cc an hour for the past two hours. She called Mr. Aguilar's physician and received an order to give Mr. Aguilar an IV diuretic. While preparing to give Mr. Aguilar the diuretic, she took his vital signs and reassessed his condition. She noted that Mr. Aguilar's skin turgor was very poor and his skin was dry. He was complaining of thirst and his blood pressure was low. Mr. Aguilar's urine was dark and concentrated in appearance. The nurse called Mr. Aguilar's physician back with this information and voiced her concern that perhaps Mr. Aguilar's low urine output was due to dehydration rather than fluid retention. Mr. Aguilar's physician ordered a urine specific gravity test, which revealed that Mr. Aguilar was in fact dehydrated. An IV diuretic could have seriously harmed Mr. Aguilar in his dehydrated condition.

▶ **EVALUATION**

- The client's fluid intake and output was accurately measured and recorded.
- Note if the client was able to participate in the recording of fluid intake and output to the best of his/her ability.
- Note and report any abnormal findings to the client's physician or qualified practitioner.

▶ **DOCUMENTATION**

Bedside Intake and Output Work Sheet

- Record all fluid I&O.
- Add totals at the end of every shift.

Intake and Output in the Medical Record

- Add totals for 24 hours.

Nurses' Notes

- Any unusual findings, excessive intake, excessive output, or serious imbalance of intake and output should be documented and reported to the patient's physician or qualified practitioner.

▶ **CRITICAL THINKING SKILL**

Introduction

Measuring and monitoring intake and output is critical to the care of a client, especially an infant.

Possible Scenario

An infant has been admitted to the pediatric unit. Her mother notes that she has been vomiting and having diarrhea. When asked, the mother was able to report how many times the baby had vomited and how many diaper changes she had performed, but she was unable to document how much fluid the baby had lost overall. The nurse admitting the baby was puzzled about how she was going to determine the baby's fluid balance baseline and how she was going to measure the baby's output. The nurse chose to use the infant's admission weight and hydration status as the baseline, ignoring the infant's current hydration status.

Possible Outcome

The infant's admission dehydration and electrolyte imbalance went untreated. The infant's status rapidly worsened, resulting in coma.

Prevention

Small children, and especially infants, are at increased risk of fluid imbalance problems. Infants have very small fluid reserves; a tablespoon of liquid is a much larger proportion of an infant's body weight than it is of an adult's. Uncontrolled diarrhea can kill infants in a matter of days. This baby girl is at risk and the nurse must be able to accurately assess the baby's fluid intake and output. The nurse can accurately assess incontinent fluid amounts by remembering how much water weighs. Weighing a diaper prior to placing it on the baby and then after it has been soiled can provide a good estimate of the amount of fluid the baby has lost. Likewise, a pad placed to catch emesis, weighed before and after use, can provide an estimate of the amount of fluid the child has vomited. It is important to remember that small children cannot tolerate fluid and electrolyte loss as well as adults. Accurate measurement and keeping the physician informed of the results are essential when caring for children.

▶ VARIATIONS

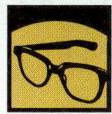

Geriatric Variations:
- *Elderly clients are sometimes incontinent. Measuring output in an incontinent client can be difficult. Weighing the client's linen or incontinence pad prior to use and then weighing it again after it has been soiled can help the caregiver keep track of the amount of fluid output the client is generating.*
- *Elderly clients need a caregiver to monitor their fluid intake, especially when they are taking diuretics, supplemental potassium, and cardiac medication.*
- *Elderly clients are at risk for fluid and electrolyte imbalances from prolonged fever or gastroenteritis.*

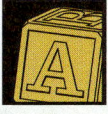

Pediatric Variations:
- *The amount of fluid loss a child can tolerate is much smaller than that of an adult because of the proportionately smaller size of the child. Small amounts of fluid loss can be serious or fatal for small children.*
- *Infants and young children are at risk for fluid and electrolyte imbalances from prolonged fever or gastroenteritis.*

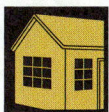

Home Care Variations:
- *The nurse should help the caregiver use standard cups and other utensils to measure intake and output.*
- *Assess the client's and caregiver's ability and compliance to record I&O.*
- *Provide appropriate charts and equipment, and teach how to record I&O.*
- *Ask the client and caregiver to perform a return demonstration for the procedure.*

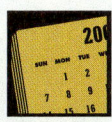

Long-Term-Care Variations:
- *Clients may suffer from a loss of appetite, including fluids.*
- *Clients may need assistance from a dietitian to prepare fluids that are appealing to them.*

▶ COMMON ERRORS

Possible Error:
Not counting the water the client drinks from the bedside pitcher.

Prevention:
Be sure the client is aware of the reasons for measuring his intake and output. Teach the client how to keep track of it. Be sure that any caregiver who is refilling water pitchers or providing juice understands the need to keep track of intake and how to do it. Teach the caregiver not to use the water in the pitcher to water flowers.

Establish a system to mark each new pitcher of water the client receives. Measure the water left in the pitcher at the end of each shift. Ask the client to help you keep track of the intake.

▶ NURSING TIPS

- Keep I&O flow sheet close to the bedside.
- Teach client's the necessity to keep accurate I&O records.
- Keep water fresh, encourage beverages as allowed.
- Record measurements immediately instead of waiting until the end of the shift.
- 240 cc ice chips equal 120 cc fluid.
- Pureed food is not considered to be fluid intake.
- Bottled nutrient tube feedings are liquid and must be considered in I&O.
- All postoperative clients are at risk for fluid loss through blood or plasma from their incision sites. Monitor the dressings.
- Remember that fluids taken to swallow pills must be recorded as intake (see Figure 1-7-7).
- Do not have visitors or family members empty bedpans, urinals, or catheter bags.

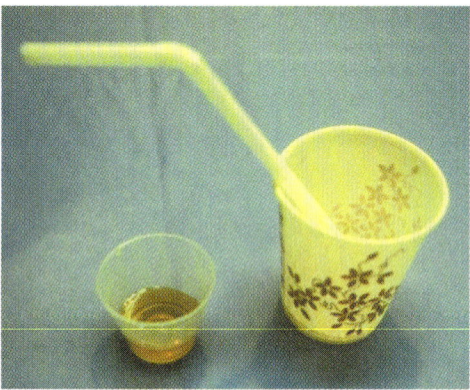

Figure 1-7-7 Even fluid used to swallow pills must be measured.

▶ SPECIAL CONSIDERATIONS

- *Proper aseptic technique should be taken when handling clients' body fluid output. Blood first, urine last. For example, if the drainage from the hemovac and urine from the urine bag need to be emptied at the same time, the health care provider should empty the hemovac first and then the urine bag and should change gloves between procedures.*
- *Infant diapers should be weighed. One gram of weight equals one cc of fluid.*

SKILL 1-8 Breast Self-Examination

Claretta Munger MSN, ARNP,
and Carla A. Bouska Lee, PhD, ARNP, FAAN

KEY TERMS

Breast assessment
Breast development
Breast examination
Cancer prevention
Chest examination
Cyst
Fibrocystic disease
Mammogram
Physical assessment of breasts
Tanner stage

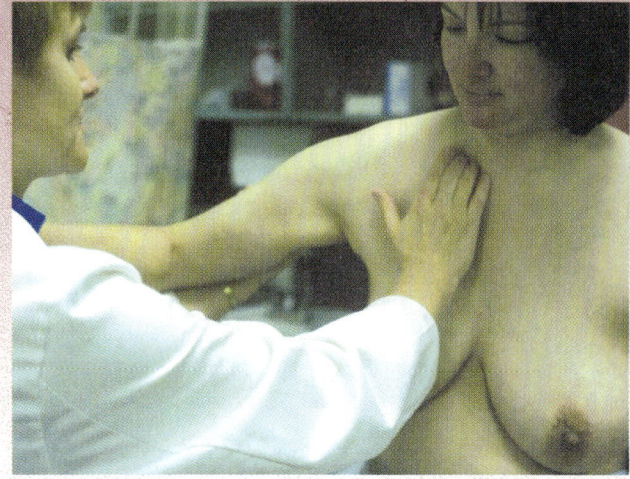

▶ OVERVIEW OF THE SKILL

Physical assessment of the breast and axillae is part of periodic health maintenance examinations for both males and females of all ages. Breast cancer cannot be prevented, but early detection offers more treatment options, and a greater chance of cure. A breast examination performed by the nurse is accompanied by breast examination education whenever possible. Teaching the client to perform monthly breast self-examinations, discussing risk factors, and prompting the client to seek recommended mammograms are essential for early diagnosis and treatment of breast cancer.

▶ ASSESSMENT

1. Assess client's musculoskeletal and range of motion ability **to determine client's ability to participate and cooperate in examination.**
2. Assess demonstrated health-seeking behaviors specific to obtaining breast examination as well as Pap and pelvic examinations **to identify any education or health-seeking deficits.**
3. Assess client's knowledge of breast self-examination and health maintenance recommendations for clinical examination **to identify further education or health-seeking deficits.**
4. Assess personal and family history relevant to cancers as well as breast and cervical abnormalities **to assist in planning health management and screening schedules.**
5. Assess if the client's health history reveals past or present use of hormonal medications, **because a thorough follow-up may be necessary if any abnormalities are found since hormonal use is a known risk factor that may increase the risk for breast cancer.**
6. Assess if the client's family history includes breast cancer in first-degree (mother or sister) or second-degree (aunt or grandmother) relatives, **because a thorough follow-up may be necessary since this is a known risk factor.**
7. Assess if the woman is postmenopausal **because breasts in postmenopausal women may show normal atrophy of glandular tissue and increased striations.**
8. Assess age for a male with enlarged breasts **because breast enlargement in adolescent males is usually normal for puberty and is common when the boy is overweight.**

81

▶ DIAGNOSIS

- Potential for Impaired Tissue Integrity.
- Health-Seeking Behaviors.
- Deficient Knowledge.

▶ PLANNING

Expected Outcomes:

1. Normal breast examination. No dimpling, nodules, masses, inflammation, lesions, discharge, lymph node enlargement, or tenderness.
2. Client is able to demonstrate proper procedure for breast self-examination and offer a plan of when it will be performed monthly.
3. Client will identify when next screening should be performed.

Equipment Needed:

- Small pillow or towel
- Centimeter ruler
- Nonsterile gloves (sterile if open lesions or drainage)
- Drape/gown
- Teaching aid for breast self-examination

▶ CLIENT EDUCATION NEEDED

1. Instruct clients not to use creams, lotions, or powders and not to shave underarms 48 hours before the scheduled assessment, because these things could alter the breast skin or cause folliculitis and lymph node enlargement.
2. Instruct clients how to prepare for and what to expect from the procedure to decrease unnecessary anxiety and to maximize cooperation.
3. Remind clients to inform you of any discomfort experienced during the procedure, because it should not be uncomfortable.
4. Teach clients to initiate breast self-examinations during puberty when they start noticing breast growth before they start menstruating. They will remember better and are interested in their bodies at this stage.
5. Teach clients to examine on an easy to remember monthly date (1st day of the month, last day of the month, the 15th, or on the day of their birth, e.g., a client born April 26th would examine on the 26th of every month) rather than in relationship to the menstrual cycle. Menses are not always regular.
6. Preventive mammograms, as recommended by age or medical history, should be scheduled as part of routine breast examination. Women need a mammogram once between the ages of 35 and 40 years and yearly after age 40. A family history of breast disease, previous abnormalities, and certain medical conditions require more frequent screening. Contact the American Cancer Society for current recommendations.
7. It is still necessary to perform monthly breast self-examinations and have a yearly clinical examination even if receiving annual mammograms. Routine self-examination will enable clients to become familiar with their normal breast tissue and identify changes.
8. Instruct clients to assess breast for lumps, dimpling, pain, nipple discharge, thickness, or any changes in breast tissue.
9. Persistent lumps should always be biopsied. Insist on a biopsy, if necessary.
10. Educate men to perform a monthly breast self-examination and obtain a clinical examination every 1–3 years, because 1% of all breast cancer is found in men.

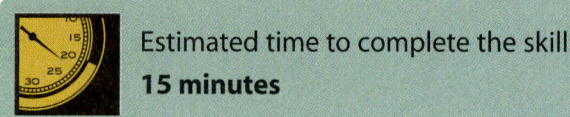

Estimated time to complete the skill: **15 minutes**

> ### ▶ DELEGATION TIPS
>
> *Breast examination and the concomitant client education skills are within the realm of the professional registered nurse's role and licensure requiring assessment and problem-solving behaviors in addition to patient teaching responsibilities. These functions must not be delegated. The ancillary personnel may reinforce the importance of breast self-examination.*

IMPLEMENTATION—ACTION/RATIONALE

ACTION	RATIONALE
1. Review personal history, medications, allergies, and family health history.	1. Identifies risk factors and previous baseline (or lack of). Identifies allergies to latex.
2. Ask the client to disrobe to the waist and to put on a gown with the opening in the front.	2. Provides easy access while maintaining maximum privacy.
3. Wash hands. Apply gloves if required by institutional policy.	3. Prevents microorganism transfer and possible contact with discharge when palpating nipples.
4. Assist the client to a sitting position facing you and expose chest and breasts (see Figure 1-8-1)	4. Allows comparison of breasts bilaterally.

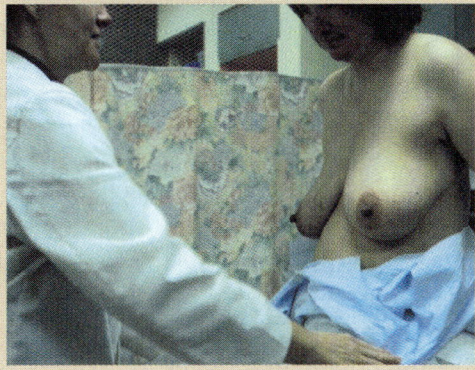

Figure 1-8-1 Assist the client to a sitting position facing the examiner.

5. Inspect breasts, areola, and nipples:

- With client's arms at sides
- With client's arms raised (see Figure 1-8-2)
- With client's hands pressed on hips (see Figure 1-8-3)
- With client's arms extended straight ahead as client leans forward (may omit this position for male unless gynecomastia is present)

5. Observe for flesh color, slight inequities in size and symmetry, rounded shape, and smooth skin surface.
   Redness, blue hue, retraction, dimpling, enlarged pores, edema, lumps, lesions, rashes, ulcers, and discharge are abnormal.
   Supernumerary nipples along the milk line are a normal variant.

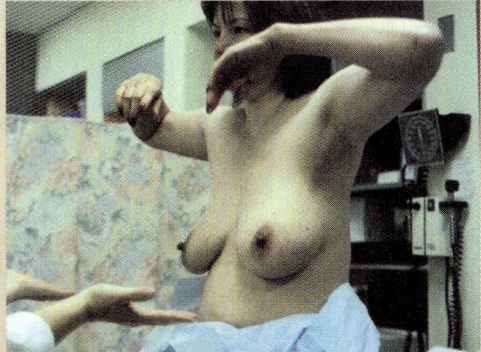

Figure 1-8-2 Inspect the breasts with the client's arms raised.

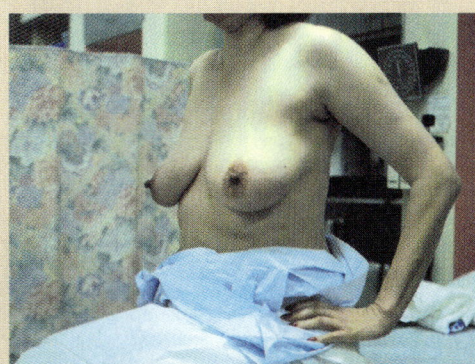

Figure 1-8-3 Inspect the breasts with the client's hands resting on hips.

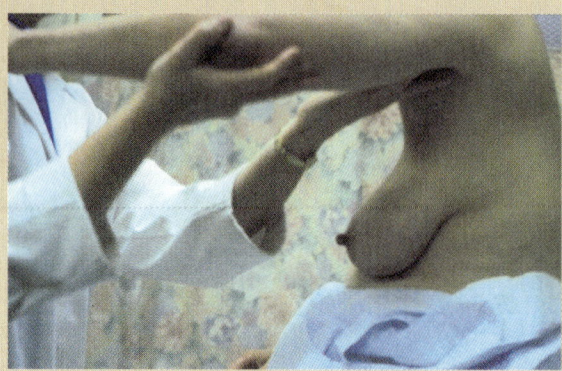

Figure 1-8-4 Palpate lymph nodes adjacent to breast tissue.

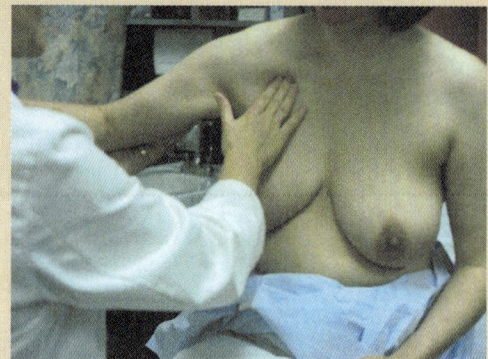

Figure 1-8-5 Palpate infraclavicular lymph nodes.

6. Palpate adjacent lymph nodes: supraclavicular, infraclavicular, and subclavian (see Figures 1-8-4 and 1-8-5).

7. Palpate breast: Using the pads of the palmar surfaces of the fingertips, palpate the right breast by gently compressing the mammary tissues against the chest wall. Palpation may be performed from the periphery to the nipple, in either concentric circles or in wedge sections (see Figure 1-8-6).

   Explain to the client and teach breast self-examination as you examine.

6. Nodes should be less than 1 cm in diameter and nontender.

7. Observe for warm temperature, elasticity, tenderness, pain, erythema, masses, or nodules, which are abnormal.

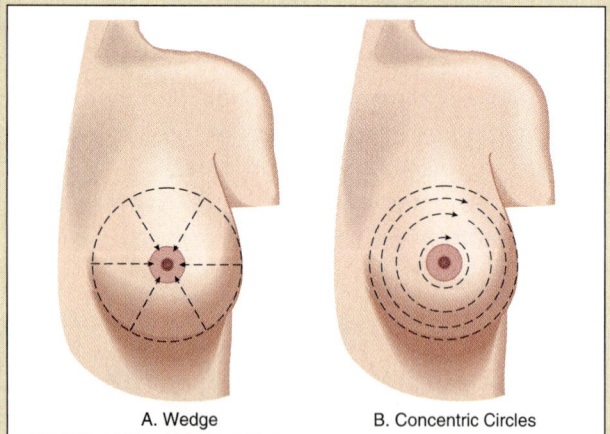

A. Wedge   B. Concentric Circles

Figure 1-8-6 Palpation methods.

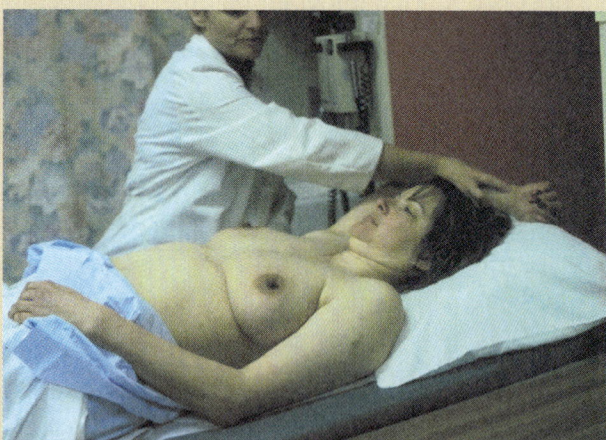

Figure 1-8-7 Place the client in a supine position.

8. Explain and teach breast self-examination as you examine. Teach the client to use the right hand to palpate the left breast and the left hand to examine the right breast. During part of the exam, place the client's fingers under the practitioner's fingers.

8. Teaching during the examination reinforces the need for and understanding of breast exams, and enables the client to identify normal breast tissue and abnormal tissue if present. Increases confidence in performing breast self-examination.

9. Palpate areola and nipple using similar circular technique as with breast. Pay special attention to subareolar area and gently press the nipple between your fingers.

10. Palpate into axilla starting at anterior axillary line and continuing at an angle to the midaxillary line and up into the axilla (using same circular fingertip motion). Have client place arm at side and palpate deep into the axilla.

11. Repeat Actions 7–9 on the left breast, areola, nipple, and axilla.

12. Assist the client to the supine position. Place arm on examination side under head and place a small pillow under the same side scapula (see Figure 1-8-7).

13. Palpate breast, areola, and nipple as in Actions 7–10 (see Figures 1-8-8 and 1-8-9).

14. Assist the client to a sitting position. Review the steps and ask the client to return demonstrate breast self-examination.

15. Allow the client to dress.

16. Remove gloves and wash hands.

17. Give the client written materials to reinforce teaching. Instruct the client when to schedule the next clinical examination.

9. Observe abnormalities such as inflammation discharge, nodules, fissuring, or lesions.

10. Identify posterior axillary, central axillary, anterior axillary, and lateral axillary node locations. Nodes should be less than 1 cm and nontender.

11. Identify normal versus abnormal as with the right breast. Compare breasts bilaterally.

12. Position spreads breast tissue over the chest wall, maximizing palpation accuracy.

13. Reevaluate examination in second position.

14. Provides more comfort for client. Evaluates success of your teaching.

15. Provides for client's comfort.

16. Reduces transmission of microorganisms.

17. Reinforces teaching. Provides a readily available form to client for reference when at home.

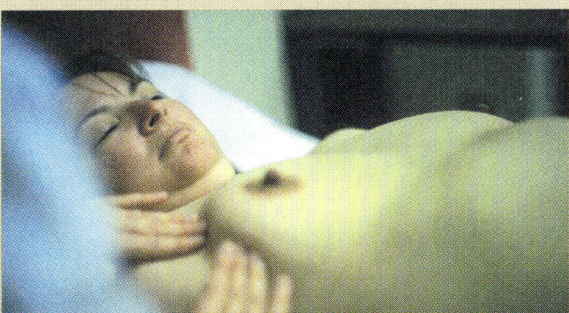

Figure 1-8-8 Palpate the breast.

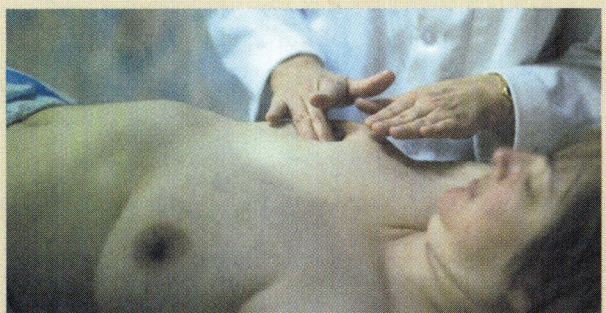

Figure 1-8-9 Palpate the areola and nipple.

REAL WORLD ANECDOTES

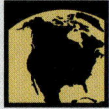

Scenario 1

Three years ago a 52-year-old woman had a bilateral mastectomy due to cancer of the right breast. She chose the bilateral mastectomy due to increased risk of an aunt having the same kind of cancer in one breast and the trauma of having to return for a second surgery after a unilateral removal. She was relieved that she no longer needed to "worry" about cancer. She quit her monthly breast self-examinations thinking that she was no longer at risk. One day she noticed it hurt as she raised her left arm. An enlarged gland was causing the discomfort. She returned to her provider and had to undergo another surgery as well as follow-up treatment. It is possible that the course of treatment could have been shortened and the success rate increased had she continued her monthly breast self-examinations and her yearly clinical examinations. She is currently undergoing treatment.

Scenario 2

Mrs. Russell talks with a nurse practitioner about a soft, oblong lump she found in her left breast. She found the lump a week ago, but she did not think it was important because it was neither round like a pea nor firm. The nurse knows that masses may not be hard and may have irregular borders. She also knows that during a breast self-examination you should be sensitive to areas in the breast that "feel different" than the rest of the breast as opposed to looking for a clearly demarcated lump. The nurse orders additional assessment.

EVALUATION

- Client is able to perform monthly breast self-examination.
- Client returns for clinical breast examination at prescribed time.
- Any abnormalities are identified early for referral evaluation and possible treatment.

DOCUMENTATION

Nurses' Notes

- Record the date and time.
- Document findings of abnormalities and absence of abnormalities.
- Record the client's response to findings and teaching.
- Record a follow-up plan, if necessary.

CRITICAL THINKING SKILL

Introduction

Ms. Hernandez, who is 30 years old, asks whether she should worry about the lumps she frequently finds in her breasts. She has a history of polycystic disease.

Possible Scenario

She ignores the lumps, attributing them to polycystic disease.

Possible Outcome

One of the lumps is not just a cyst; it is malignant.

Prevention

Advise the client to never ignore lumps or diagnose them herself. She should continue monthly breast self-examinations and, at a minimum, have a yearly clinical exam. She should report any new or changed lumps to her primary provider and ask for an assessment no matter how many times the tests show a lump is benign.

▶ VARIATIONS

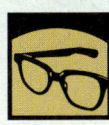

Geriatric Variations:
- Breasts are less firm, more pendulous, and often atrophied. The tissue is more coarse and more nodular.
- Be sure to lift pendulous breasts to inspect the skin under the breasts. This is a frequent site of yeast infection and needs immediate treatment. Do not use cornstarch to dry this area because cornstarch promotes yeast growth.
- Striae are normal with aging.

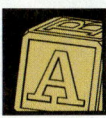

Pediatric Variations:
- At puberty when breast development starts, breasts are frequently asymmetrical.
- Overweight adolescents often falsely appear to have gynecomastia, especially during the prepubescent increase in adipose tissue.
- Inverted nipples are "normal" variants.
- Infants may have nipple discharge and up to 2 cm breast tissue from maternal estrogens.

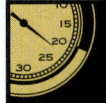

Pregnancy Variations:
- Striae are common during pregnancy and sometimes after pregnancy if breasts remain large.
- Enlargement, tingling, tenderness, increased vascularity, increased alveoli, nodularity, darkening of the areolae, and erect and sensitive nipples are common during pregnancy.
- Lactation may occur prior to delivery. Colostrum may be secreted beginning in the second trimester (week 16).
- Note if nipples are inverted, because this requires more teaching if breastfeeding is planned.

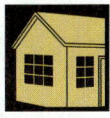

Home Care Variations:
- Teach a caregiver or family member the breast self-examination procedure if the client is unable to perform own examination.
- Omit certain positions, if necessary, for clients with medical conditions that limit movement or balance.
- If a client is rarely out of bed, teach the client or a caregiver to perform the breast self-examination when the client is both sitting up in a chair and lying in bed.

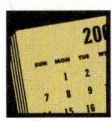

Long-Term-Care Variations:
- Omit certain positions, if necessary, for clients with medical conditions that limit movement or balance.
- If a client is rarely out of bed, the nurse or caregiver can perform the breast self-examination when the client is sitting up in a chair or lying in bed.

▶ COMMON ERRORS

Possible Error:

Breast self-examination was stopped after no lumps were detected using the first two positions. An existing lump was not detected.

Prevention:

Never assume that no detection of lumps in the first few positions means you will find nothing in the remaining positions. Do not rush the examination.

Carefully explain each step and substep to the client. It is important for the client to understand the importance of every step so she can perform breast self-examinations and receive follow-up screening.

Possible Error:

Client does not understand how to correctly perform breast self-examination.

Prevention:

It is important for the client to understand the importance of every step so she can perform regular breast self-examinations and receive follow-up screening.

▶ NURSING TIPS

- Breast examinations vary. Many practitioners use the "roll" method whereby the examiner's hands never leave the breast. Finger pads roll back and forth across the breast from the sternum to the axillae and advance an inch with each forward motion. In this method all areas of the breast are examined.
- Special attention should be given to the area under and surrounding the nipple and in the upper outer quadrant, because most lumps are found in these locations.
- Putting on gloves prior to palpation often makes the client more comfortable, because it adds an element of depersonalization.
- To reinforce self-examination, use the same circular examination techniques recommended for breast self-examination, but a wedge or vertical pattern may be used as well. It is often helpful to use these alternate techniques to reexamine any abnormalities you find. It does not alarm the client as much.
- Use the flat pads of three fingers to palpate the breast tissue by compressing it gently against the breast wall.
- Use a bimanual palpation technique in large and/or pendulous breasts.
- Usually if you explain exactly what you are doing and what you are looking for as you examine, there are no misunderstandings. If you are at all uncomfortable performing an examination, ask a "witness" to assist you to be sure that the client does not misinterpret your actions as inappropriate. With children, have the parent witness your examination.
- Expose only the area(s) being examined without undue exposure of other areas. For example, expose both breasts for inspection to compare bilaterally and then cover one breast while you palpate the other.
- Breasts are not always symmetrical. Always review breast development in light of Tanner's sexual maturity ratings (see Table 1-8-1). Correlate this with genital development whenever possible.
- Refer all abnormal or questionable findings. Describe nodules and masses as to number, shape, consistency, definition, mobility, tenderness, and skin retraction.

Table 1-8-1 Sexual Maturity Rating for Female Breast Development

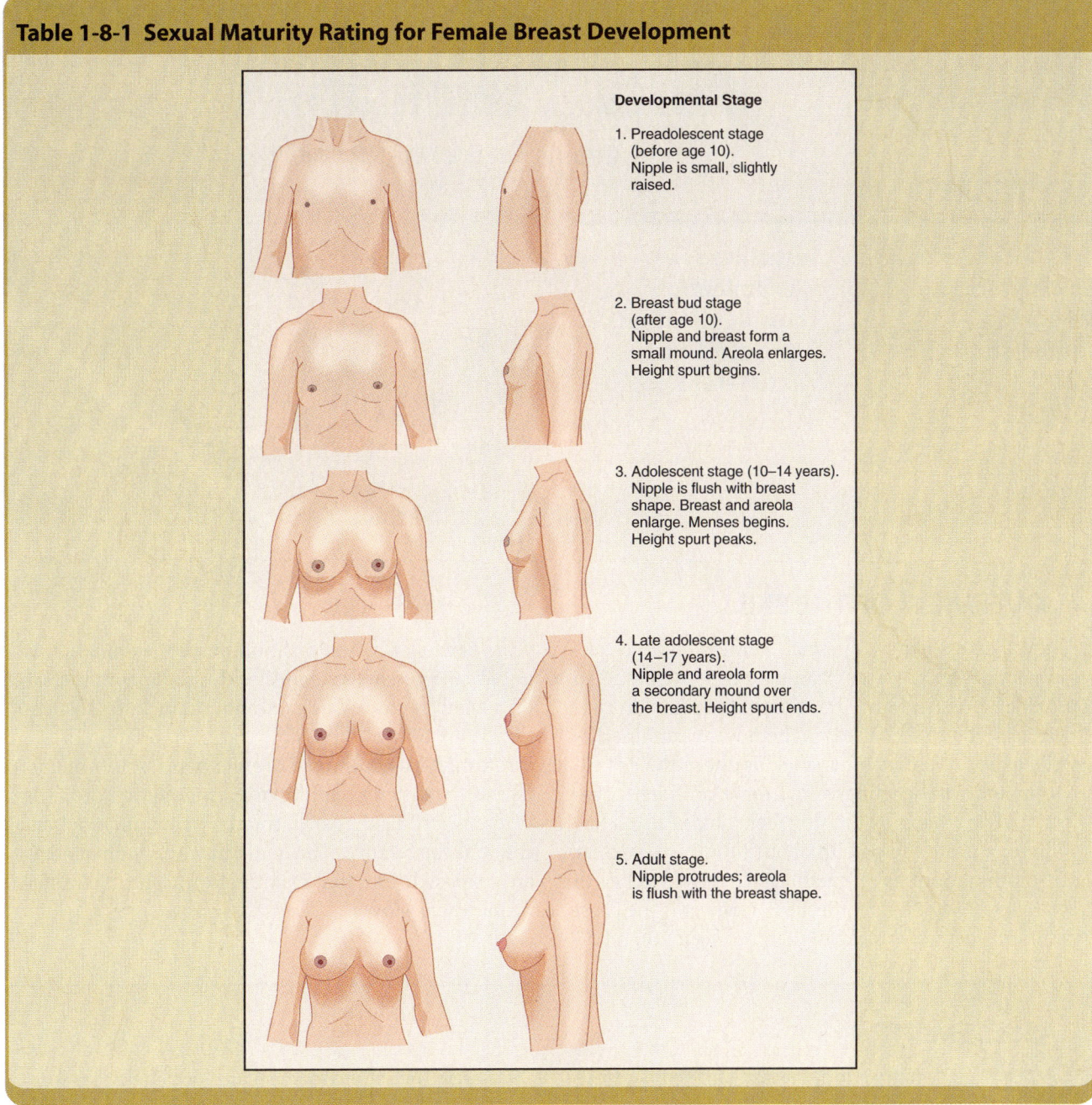

Data from *Health Assessment: Physical Examination*, Second Edition by M.E. Zator-Estes, 2002, Clifton Park, NY: Delmar Learning. Copyright 2002 by Delmar Thomson Learning.

▶ SPECIAL CONSIDERATIONS

- Women who have had breast surgery still need clinical and monthly breast self-examination to the chest, clavicle, axillae, and incision areas.
- Women with a history of fibrocystic breast may require more instructional time to identify their normal breast tissue.
- Men require breast examination, especially those with gynecomastia or on hormonal treatment.
- Heavy caffeine or chocolate consumption may cause breast pain.

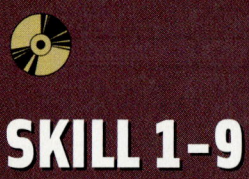

SKILL 1-9

Male Genitalia, Hernia, and Rectal Examination

Eileen M. Collins, RN, MN, ARNP, CNOR

KEY TERMS

Cremaster reflex
Epididymis
Smegma
Tanner stage
Testicular self-examination
Transillumination of the scrotum
Vas deferens

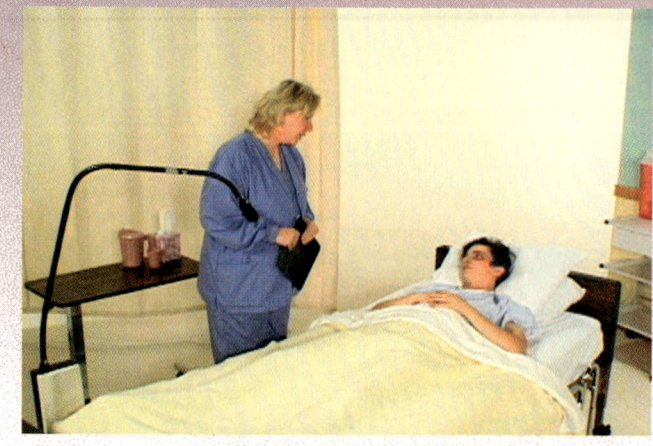

▶ OVERVIEW OF THE SKILL

Physical assessment of the male genitalia is an essential part of the physical examination. It is helpful to provide a private, warm examining area where the patient is made to feel at ease. The novice examiner, as well as the patient, is often anxious about the examination and will benefit greatly from a confident, professional approach by the provider. This is also a key time to educate the patient about monthly testicular self-examination as a method to enhance health awareness and self-care. (Testicular cancer is the most common form of cancer in men between 20 and 35 years of age.) The best position for the examination is to have the gowned patient stand and the examiner sit on a chair or stool. The examination includes inspection, palpation, and possibly transillumination of the scrotum. Areas examined are the penis, scrotum and its contents, testis, epididymis, spermatic cord, vas deferens within the cord, inguinal ring, inguinal areas, and the rectum. The genitalia and inguinal areas are exposed for the examination. The examiner should wear gloves.

▶ ASSESSMENT

1. Assess sexual maturation, the size and shape of the penis, the skin integrity to include erythema or discolorations, swelling, or lesions.
2. Note the color and texture of the scrotal skin as well as the character and distribution of pubic hair. Note size, contour, and symmetry.
3. Tanner stage for children and adolescents.
4. Assess testicular size and adnexal structures.
5. Inspect the inguinal areas and groin for nodules, swelling, or bulges.
6. Assess the cremaster reflex.
7. Assess the prostate gland for size, shape, consistency, sensitivity, and mobility of the prostate.
8. Assess the seminal vesicles for tenderness and masses.
9. Assess the sacrococcygeal and perianal areas for lumps, lesions, inflammation, excoriations, and tenderness.
10. Assess rectal sphincter tone and palpate for nodules, tenderness, induration, or irregularities of the rectal surface.

▶ DIAGNOSIS

- Potential for Impaired Tissue Integrity.
- Health-Seeking Behaviors.
- Deficient Knowledge.
- Anxiety. The patient may have anxiety related to the nature of the exam.

SKILL 1-9 Male Genitalia, Hernia, and Rectal Examination

▶ PLANNING

Expected Outcomes:

1. Normal penile exam. No erythema or discolorations, swelling, or lesions.
2. Normal exam of the scrotum, with normal size, contour, and symmetry.
3. Tanner stage is appropriate for age.
4. Testicular size and adnexal structures are within normal limits.
5. Inguinal areas and groin are free of nodules, swelling, and bulges.
6. The prostate gland is within normal limits for size, shape, consistency, sensitivity, and mobility.

Equipment Needed:

- Gloves (clean)
- Flashlight for transillumination
- Lubricant for rectal exam

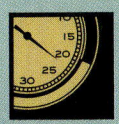

Estimated time to complete the skill: **15–20 minutes**

▶ CLIENT EDUCATION NEEDED

1. Instruct the client on how to prepare for the examination and what to expect to decrease unnecessary anxiety and to illicit cooperation.
2. Remind the client to inform you of any discomfort experienced during the exam.
3. Teach and encourage monthly testicular self-examination.

▶ DELEGATION TIPS

Testicular examination and the concomitant client education are skills within the realm of the professional Registered Nurse's role and licensure, requiring assessment and problem-solving behaviors in addition to client teaching. These functions must not be delegated. The ancillary personnel may reinforce the importance of testicular self-examination. During the provision of personal hygiene to a male client the ancillary personnel must note and report any abnormalities of the genitalia, such as unusual odors, discharge, or edema.

IMPLEMENTATION—ACTION/RATIONALE

ACTION	RATIONALE
Penile Examination	
1. Ask the client to disrobe completely and to put on a gown.	1. Provides easy access for the exam.
2. Explain the procedure to the client (see Figure 1-9-1).	2. Decreases the client's anxiety level.
3. Wash hands, and apply clean gloves.	3. Practice clean technique.
4. Have the client stand and hold up his gown to expose the genitalia.	4. Provides best exposure for examination.

continues

Penile examination continued

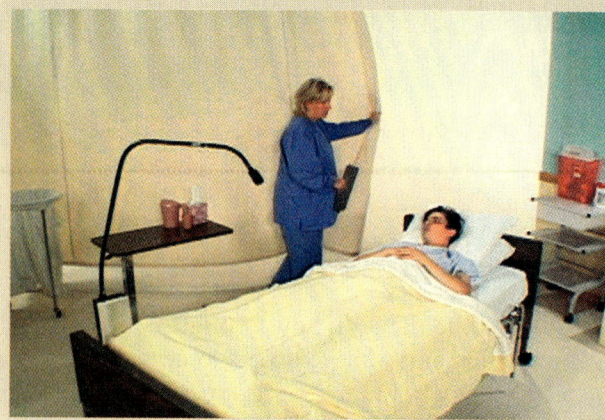

Figure 1-9-1 Provide for the client's privacy, and explain the procedure.

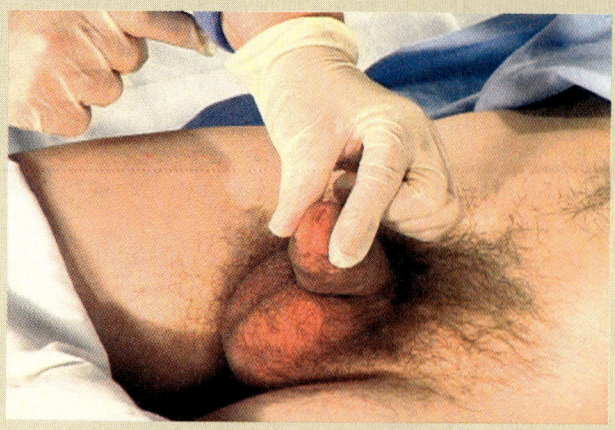

Figure 1-9-2 Inspect the glans penis and urethral meatus.

5. Inspect the penis and pubic hair distribution. Check the skin at the base of the penis for rash, lesions, nits, or lice.

6. Retract, or have the client retract, the prepuce (foreskin), if present.

7. Observe the glans penis and the urethral meatus. Open the urethral meatus by compressing the glans gently between your index finger above and thumb below. Note the location of the urethral meatus as well as any discharge, ulcers, scars, nodules, lesions, or signs of inflammation.

8. Palpate the entire length of the penis between your thumb and the first two fingers (see Figure 1-9-3).

5. Tanner stage in boys; note size, color, integrity (lesions, rash, pustules).

6. The uncircumcised male will have foreskin over the glans, which should be easily retracted. It is necessary to retract the prepuce to detect chancres or carcinoma. Smegma, a cheesy secretion, may accumulate normally under the foreskin.

7. The skin of the glans penis should be smooth and without ulceration. The urethral meatus is normally located ventrally on the end of the penis. There is normally no discharge. If discharge is present, obtain a culture for gonorrhea and Chlamydia (see Figure 1-9-2).

8. Note any tenderness, induration, or masses.
   Palpation of the shaft may be omitted in a young, asymptomatic client.
   Replace the foreskin, if retracted, before continuing with the exam.

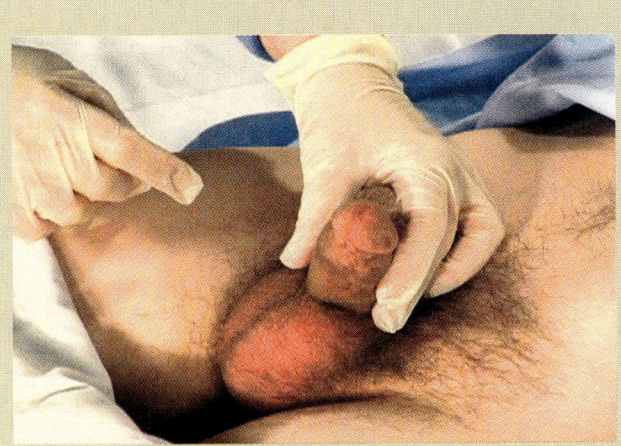 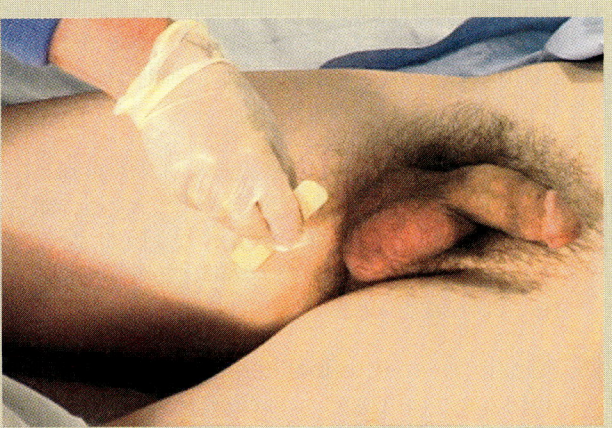

Figure 1-9-3 Use the thumb and first two fingers to palpate the entire length of the penis.

Figure 1-9-4 Elicit the cremaster reflex.

Scrotal Examination

9. Inspect the scrotum for erythema, discoloration, swelling, and skin integrity.

9. Abnormalities in the scrotum can be indicative of local trauma, inflammation, hernias, or systemic conditions, such as heart or renal failure.

10. Elicit the cremaster reflex on both sides (see Figure 1-9-4).

10. Absence of this reflex may be the most sensitive physical finding for torsion of the testicle. It is performed by gently stroking or pinching the superior medial aspect of the thigh, resulting in brisk ipsilateral testicular torsion or retraction.

11. Palpate each testis and epididymis between the thumb and first two fingers. Note their size, lie (high or low within the scrotum), shape, consistency, and tenderness.

    The length of a normal testis should be greater than 4 cm and the volume greater than 20 ml.

    Testicular Torsion is a Surgical Emergency.

11. The left testicle normally sits slightly lower than the right testicle. The testicles are rubbery and approximately equal in size.

    Pressure on the testis normally produces a deep visceral pain.

    Twisting or torsion of the testis causes venous obstruction, edema, and eventually arterial obstruction (rarely seen over the age of 20–30 years). It is a significant cause of sterility and morbidity in men.

12. Palpate each spermatic cord, including the vas deferens within the cord, between your thumb and fingers from the epididymis to the inguinal ring. Note any nodules or swelling.

12. Any swelling in the scrotum should be evaluated by transillumination. Shine a beam of light (flashlight) from behind the scrotum through the mass. Normal testis do not transilluminate. Look for transmission of light as a red glow: swellings that contain serous fluid (hydrocele, spermatocele) transilluminate.

Hernia examination

13. Inspect the inguinal and femoral areas. Ask the client to strain down or cough while you continue your observation.

14. Palpate for a **femoral** hernia by placing your fingers on the anterior thigh in the region of the femoral canal. Ask the client to bear down or cough as you note any palpable masses, tenderness, or swelling.

15. Palpate for an **inguinal** hernia. Using your right hand for the client's right side and your left hand for the client's left side, just above the testicle, invaginate the loose scrotal skin with your index finger. Follow the spermatic cord upward to find a triangular slit-like opening of the external inguinal ring. If the inguinal ring is enlarged enough to admit your finger, then gently follow the inguinal canal and ask the client to cough. Note any herniating mass felt against the finger.

Rectal Examination

16. Position the client for ease of examination.

13. A bulge that presents on straining suggests a hernia.

14. Small (1.0 cm), freely mobile lymph nodes may normally be found in the inguinal area (see Figure 1-9-5).

15. If present, a herniating mass will generally be felt against the side of the finger (see Figure 1-9-6).

16. If the client is standing after the completion of the genital examination, have him bend and lean on the exam table, with legs slightly apart, exposing the rectum to the examiner. Or,
    Ask the client to lie in a left lateral decubitus position, on his left side, placing his buttocks close to the edge of the table nearest the examiner. Flex the client's hips and knees to stabilize the client and improve visibility.

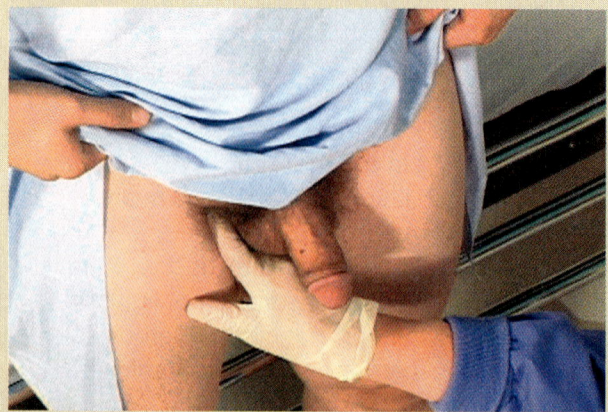

Figure 1-9-5 Palpate for a femoral hernia.

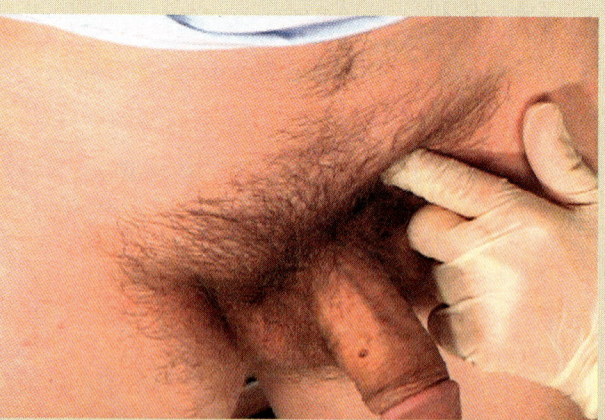

Figure 1-9-6 Palpate for an inguinal hernia.

17. Provide a warm, quiet environment with appropriate lighting. Drape the client so that only his buttocks are exposed. Explain the procedure to the client.

17. Decreases the client's anxiety and provides privacy. Gentle, slow movement of the examiner's finger accompanied by explanation and a calm demeanor will ensure a successful exam.

18. Wash hands, and apply clean gloves.

18. This is a clean procedure.

19. Spread apart the buttocks and examine the anus, perianal area, and sacral region for any scars, lesions, nodules, inflammation, ulcerations, or abnormalities. Ask the client to bear down as you assess for any bulges (see Figure 1-9-7).

19. Adult perianal skin is normally more pigmented and coarser than the skin over the buttocks.
    As the client strains down, note any tissue protrusion or hemorrhoids. Reassure the client that sensations of urination and defecation are normal.

20. Lubricate the gloved index finger. As the client strains down, rest the pad of the finger over the anus. As the sphincter relaxes, slowly insert the finger into the anal canal, with the finger facing the umbilicus. Note sphincter tone and any masses, nodules, or tenderness.

20. The anal canal is approximately 2.5 cm long. It is bordered by the external and internal anal sphincters, which normally are firm and smooth.

21. Insert the finger as far as possible into the rectum. Rotate your hand to palpate the walls of the rectum laterally and posteriorly while rotating your index finger.

21. The wall of the rectum should be smooth and moist.

22. Anteriorally palpate the two lobes of the prostate gland and its sulcus. Note the size, shape, and consistency of the prostate as you identify any irregularities, such as nodules, masses, or tenderness.

22. Inform the client that he may feel the urge to urinate when you examine the prostate, that this is a normal sensation, and that he will not void.
    The male prostate gland is approximately 2.5 cm long. It is smooth, nonmovable, nontender, and rubbery to the touch.

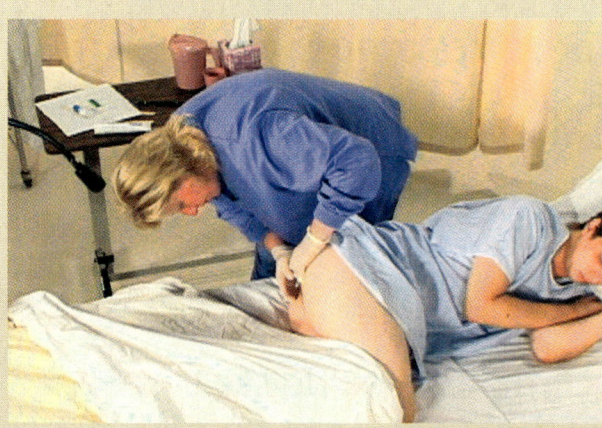

Figure 1-9-7 Left dorsal positioning for rectal examination.

continues

Rectal Examination *continued*

23. If possible, extend your finger above the prostate region and palpate the superior portion of the lateral lobe, to the region of the seminal vesicles and the peritoneal cavity.

24. Gently withdraw your finger. Note the color of any fecal material on your glove and test for occult blood.

25. Offer the client tissues or wipe excess lubricant/stool from the anus.

23. The seminal vesicles are not normally palpable unless swollen. Note nodules, cysts, or tenderness.

24. There is normally no occult blood in the stools.

25. Provide for client comfort.

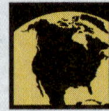

▶ **REAL WORLD ANECDOTES**

*Mr. Amin is a 35-year-old Somalian who presents to the clinic complaining of a swollen right testicle. It causes him pain when he turns his foot out to the side and when he bends over. He states that he is sexually active and usually uses condoms during coitus. On examination, his right testicle is enlarged and tender. His epididymis also is very tender on this side. You obtain a culture from the meatal opening and send it to the lab. Then you get a urine sample for culture and sensitivity testing. It is important to get the culture from the penis **before** you get the urine culture, because the urine will wash away the specimen needed for a diagnosis of Chlamydia. You treat Mr. Amin for Chlamydia and give him information about preventing sexually transmitted diseases.*

▶ **EVALUATION**

- Any abnormalities are identified early for treatment and/or referral evaluation.
- The client is able to perform monthly testicular self-examinations.
- The client returns to his health care provider for regular checkups.

▶ **DOCUMENTATION**

- Record the date and time of the examination.
- Include the client's physiological findings of abnormalities and absence of abnormalities.
- Record the client's response to the findings.
- Document instruction and return demonstration of testicular self-examination.
- Record a follow-up plan, if necessary.

▶ **CRITICAL THINKING SKILL**

Introduction

Mr. Gomez, an African-American 50-year-old laborer, states he has discovered a lump in his testicle. He has not had a prostate exam since he was 40 years old, and he was fine at that time.

Possible Scenario

He ignores the lump as a normal sign of aging.

Possible Outcome

The lump may be a malignancy from prostate cancer.

Prevention

Advise Mr. Gomez never to disregard a lump. He should report it to his health care provider immediately. Commend him for performing self-testicular exams, and encourage him to have yearly clinical examinations. African-American men are at increased risk for prostate cancer and should be screened regularly with PSA testing and digital rectal examination.

SKILL 1-9 Male Genitalia, Hernia, and Rectal Examination

▶ VARIATIONS

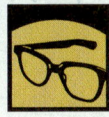

Geriatric Variations:
- The external genitalia reveals thinner, sometimes gray, pubic hair.
- The penis decreases in size, and the testicles may appear small or atrophied as they hang lower in the scrotum.
- Testosterone production and secretion decrease with age; however, serum levels may be in the low-normal range through the age of 80 years.
- The ability to attain an erection may be delayed, and full erection is not always possible.
- The elderly male might note a reduction or absence in preejaculatory fluid emission. Advise sexually active older men that spermatogenesis may continue into advanced age.

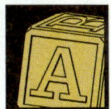

Child Care Variation:
- Check for sexual maturity rating in boys by using the Tanner Staging criteria. A noticeable increase in the size of the testes, usually between the ages of 9.5 and 13.5 years, is a sign of initiation of puberty. Next, pubic hair begins to grow and the penis increases in size. The change from preadolescent to adult takes about 3 years, with a range from less than 2 years to almost 5 years.

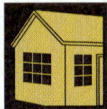

Home Care Variation:
- If a patient is disabled, he may not be able to perform testicular self-examination. He may need a health care provider to do and relay any significant findings to the physician.

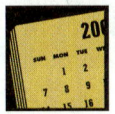

Long-term Care Variations:
- Urinary retention and incontinence may occur related to prostatic changes in the elderly. It is imperative to provide yearly checkups and testicular self-examination in this population.

▶ COMMON ERRORS

Possible error:

The client presented with an enlarged scrotum and urinary frequency and was asked for a urine sample.

Prevention:

With a male client, always obtain the urine specimen **after** the physical examination because a sample from the urinary meatus may be needed. When Chlamydia is suspected, the meatus must be swabbed for a culture. Urination washes away the sample and should be deferred until the culture is taken.

▶ NURSING TIPS

- If a large scrotal mass is found, ask the client to lie down for further examination. If the mass returns to the abdomen, a hernia is confirmed. If you can get your fingers above the mass in the scrotum, then a hydrocele is suspected. Listen to the mass with a stethoscope. Bowel sounds can be heard over a hernia but not over a hydrocele.

- When the uncircumcised male client is examined, the foreskin must be retracted for a thorough examination. This prepuce must be returned its normal position after the examination to prevent injury to the client.

▶ SPECIAL CONSIDERATIONS

- *When a client presents with testicular torsion, the history may reveal a minor similar pain in the past that resolved spontaneously. Clients usually present with sudden onset of severe, unilateral scrotal pain that may be associated with nausea and vomiting. Scrotal edema and erythema as well as abdominal pain may occur.*
- *According to the American Urological Association, African-American men and men with a first-degree relative with prostate cancer should be evaluated with annual PSA testing and rectal examination beginning at 40 years of age. All other men should have an initial evaluation at 50 years of age.*

SKILL 1-10

Collecting a Clean-Catch, Midstream Urine Specimen

Carla A. Bouska Lee, PhD, ARNP, FAAN,
and Gaylene Bouska Altman, RN, PhD

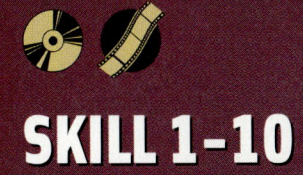

KEY TERMS

Clean-catch specimen
Clean-voided specimen
Midstream specimen
Specimen
Urine specimen

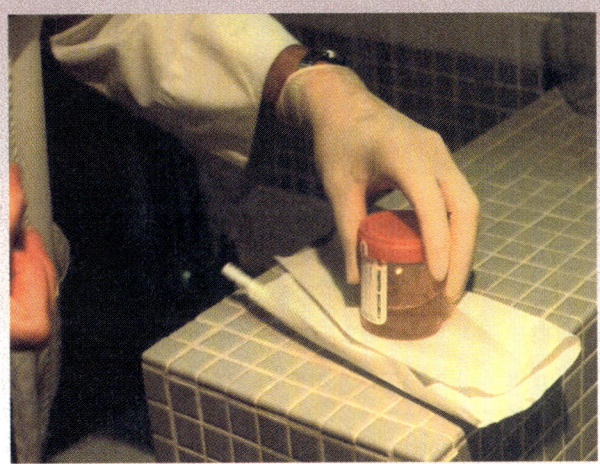

▶ OVERVIEW OF THE SKILL

A clean urine specimen to be used for culture and sensitivity can be collected without using an invasive method such as catheterization. This procedure is referred to as a clean-voided, clean-catch, or midstream urine specimen in that it is not a sterile procedure such as catheterization but, rather, a method of obtaining a clean specimen. This procedure is best accomplished with the client on the toilet because the use of a urinal or bedpan increases the risk of contamination. The client is asked to clean himself and initiate urination. After the client starts voiding, a sterile collection cup is placed under the stream of urine and a specimen collected. Hence it is called midstream collection. The initial urine is not collected because this portion of the stream flushes the urethral opening and meatus of any bacteria. The end urine is not collected because as the urine stream slows, and increased dripping and contact with the meatus occurs, the chance of contamination increases. The clean-catch specimen is sent to a laboratory for analysis.

▶ ASSESSMENT

1. Evaluate the client's ability to obtain a clean-catch specimen to **determine if the client is able to clean himself appropriately and understands the need to obtain a midstream specimen.**
2. Assess the presence of signs and symptoms of urinary tract infections or other abnormalities **because burning or the inability to control urination may hamper the client's ability to obtain a clean specimen.**

▶ DIAGNOSIS

- Impaired Urinary Elimination.
- Pain, related to potential urinary tract infection.
- Deficient Knowledge, related to personal hygiene.
- Disturbed Body Image.

CHAPTER 1   Physical Assessment

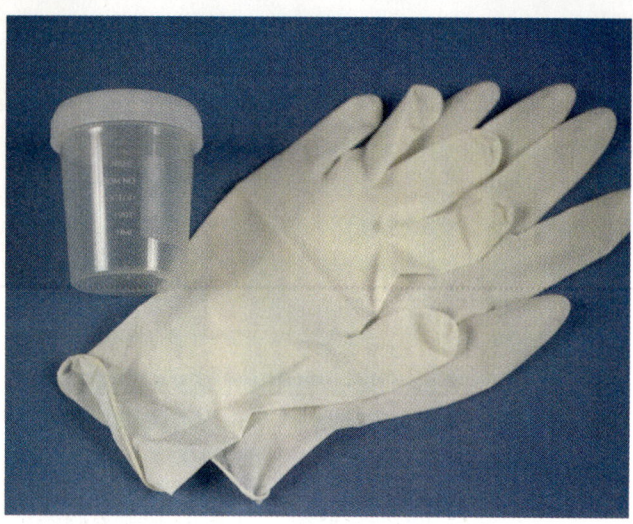

Figure 1-10-1 Sterile specimen cup and gloves.

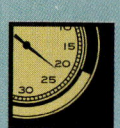 Estimated time to complete the skill: **10–15 minutes**

Equipment Needed (see Figure 1-10-1):
- Sterile collection container with lid and label
- Sterile midstream kit, antiseptic towelettes, or cotton balls with antiseptic solution
- Toilet paper
- Nonsterile gloves
- Sterile gauze (optional)

▶ PLANNING

Expected Outcomes:
1. Client will be able to obtain a clean, midstream specimen.
2. Client will have absence of urinary abnormalities, such as burning, tingling, pain upon urination, or inability to control stream.
3. Client will understand procedure.

▶ CLIENT EDUCATION NEEDED

1. Instruct clients regarding need for clean, noncontaminated, specimen.
2. Instruct clients how to collect specimen, open kit or towelettes, and use antiseptic solutions.
3. Instruct clients regarding need for procedure.

▶ DELEGATION TIP

Collection of a clean-catch specimen may be delegated to ancillary personnel properly trained in the technique of cleaning the patient and obtaining the voided specimen.

IMPLEMENTATION—ACTION/RATIONALE

ACTION	RATIONALE
1. Check orders and assess need for the procedure.	1. Provides understanding of the purpose of the procedure.
2. Gather equipment.	2. Provides for organization.
3. Assess the client's ability to complete the procedure, including understanding, mobility, and balance.	3. Improves compliance and likelihood of obtaining sterile specimen.
4. Assess the client for signs and symptoms of urinary abnormalities.	4. Improves compliance and provides baseline data.
5. Check the client's identification.	5. Ensures accuracy.

SKILL 1-10 Collecting a Clean-Catch, Midstream Urine Specimen

6. If the client is to complete the procedure in privacy, explain the procedure, give equipment to the client, and wait for specimen. If the client has decreased personal hygiene, perform the procedure after a bath or have the client wash the perineal area before a procedure.

6. Increases compliance. Protects client from embarrassment.

7. If the nurse is to perform the procedure: Wash hands and apply gloves. If the client is to perform the procedure, instruct the client to wash hands before and after the procedure. If the client is more comfortable, allow him/her to wear gloves.

7. Decreases transmission of microorganisms.

8. Provide privacy.

8. Decreases embarrassment.

9. Instruct the client. Female client: Sit with legs separated on the toilet. Male client: Sit down to help control splashing.

9. Increases compliance and understanding.

10. Using sterile procedure, open kit or towelettes (see Figure 1-10-2). Open sterile container, placing the lid with sterile side up on a firm surface (see Figure 1-10-3).

10. Prevents contamination of the specimen.

11. Use the thumb and forefinger to separate the labia, or have the client separate the labia with fingers (see Figure 1-10-4).

11. Provides access for cleaning the labia.

12. Female client: With the labia separated, use a downward stroke (from the top of the labia down toward the rectal area), and cleanse one side of the labia with the towelette (see Figure 1-10-5).
    Discard the towelette and repeat the procedure on the other side with another

12. Cleanses area and prevents contamination of clean area. Prevents contamination by feces. Keeping labia separated avoids contamination and decreases microorganisms in specimen.

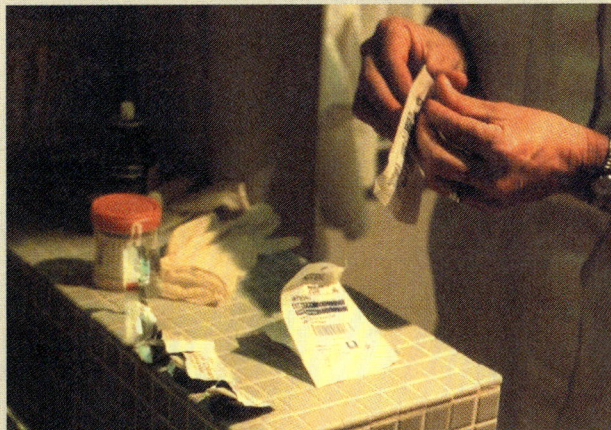

Figure 1-10-2 Open specimen cup and kit or cleansing towel packages prior to beginning the procedure.

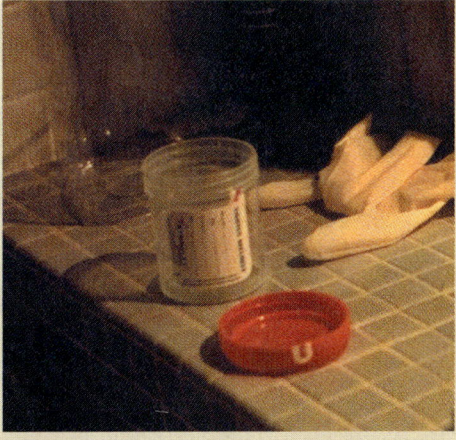

Figure 1-10-3 Place the lid on a firm surface, sterile side up. Do not touch the inside of the lid.

continues

102 CHAPTER 1 Collecting a Clean-Catch, Midstream Urine Specimen

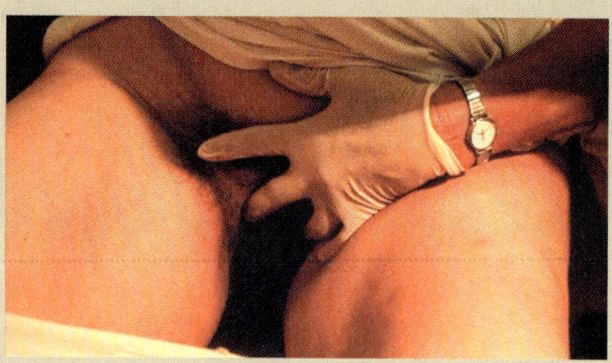

Figure 1-10-4 Separate the labia with the fingers of the nondominant hand.

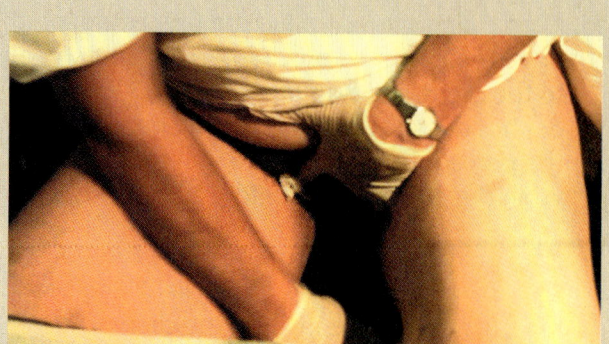

Figure 1-10-6 Place the specimen cup under the urine stream.

towelette, keeping the labia separated at all times. With a third towelette, use a downward stroke from the top of the urethral opening to the bottom. Discard the towelette.

Male client: Pull back the foreskin (if present in uncircumcised male) and clean with a single stroke around meatus and glans. Use a circular motion starting with the head of the penis at the urethral opening, moving down the glans shaft. Discard the towelette and repeat the procedure with another towelette, keeping the foreskin retracted. Cleanse the head of the penis three times using a circular motion. Use a new towelette each time.

Prevents contamination of microorganisms from foreskin. Single strokes and moving away from opening prevents contamination of the urethral opening.

13. Ask the client to begin to urinate into the toilet. After the stream starts with good flow, place the collection cup under the stream of urine. Avoid touching the skin with the container. Fill the container with 30–60 cc of urine and remove the container before urination ceases (see Figure 1-10-6). Wipe with toilet paper.

13. The specimen is collected midstream to avoid contamination of urine that touches the labia. The initial urine flushes bacteria from the orifice and the end urine may have contact with the meatus or labia and, hence, be contaminated.

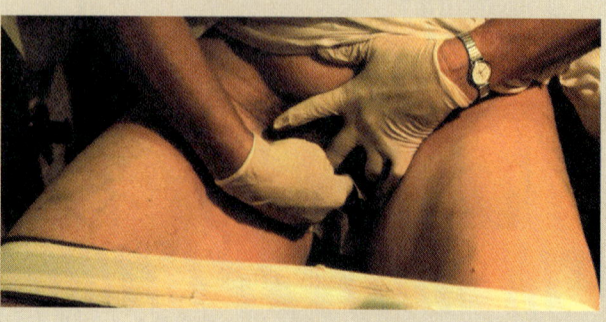

Figure 1-10-5 Cleanse each side and down the middle using a single downward stroke for each towelette. Keep the labia separated.

SKILL 1-10 Collecting a Clean-Catch, Midstream Urine Specimen

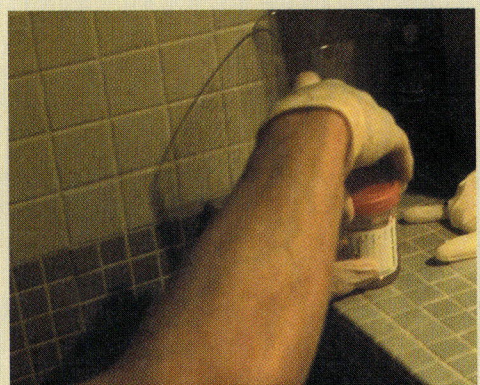

Figure 1-10-7   Replace the lid and close tightly.

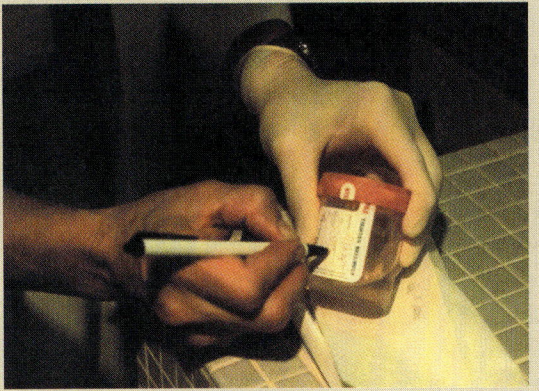

Figure 1-10-8   Label the container with the client, date, and time the specimen was collected.

14. Place the sterile lid back onto the container and close tightly (see Figure 1-10-7).
    Clean and dry the outside of the container with a towelette. Wash hands. Label and enclose in a plastic biohazard bag (see Figure 1-10-8), and follow facility policy for transporting specimen to the laboratory.

14. Prevents contamination of sterile specimen, prevents spillage, and ensures accuracy.

15. Remove and dispose of gloves and wash hands.

15. Decreases transmission of microorganisms.

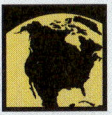 ▶ **REAL WORLD ANECDOTES**

Mr. Alvarez, 65 years old, is asked by a physician's assistant to provide a urine specimen. The nurse gives him a container and instructions on how to obtain a sterile clean-catch specimen. Mr. Alvarez is afraid he will not be able to produce enough urine if he waits for a midstream collection so he places the cup prior to beginning urination. When he returns the filled specimen cup, the nurse asks him if he followed her instructions. He admits that he did not get the sample midstream. The nurse explains the importance of following the procedure to obtain a sterile sample. Mr. Alvarez is asked to return after lunch.

▶ **EVALUATION**

- Evaluate characteristics of urine.
- Evaluate client's compliance.
- Evaluate client's complaints associated with urination, such as burning, pain, or inability to initiate urination.

▶ **DOCUMENTATION**

Nurses' Notes

- Document procedure.
- Document characteristics of urine.
- Document client's signs and symptoms associated with urination.

▶ **CRITICAL THINKING SKILL**

Introduction

Helping a client overcome embarrassment can prevent an invasive procedure.

Possible Scenario

A client came into the emergency room at 2:30 AM with a fever of 102.3°F, complaining of bloody urine, dizziness, chills, and pelvic pain. The physician ordered a clean-catch urine specimen. The client was given a sterile specimen cup and ordered to go into the bathroom and return with the sample immediately, because the lab courier was waiting. At the front counter, with several staff and family members within earshot, the nurse gave the client instructions on how to clean herself and void.

Possible Outcome

Embarrassed by the request to void on demand, and the thought that several people knew she was in the bathroom voiding, the client was not able to void. The nurse was unable to collect a specimen. After several attempts, the physician ordered the client catheterized to obtain a sterile sample.

Prevention

Increase fluids. Provide both visual and auditory privacy for client education. Assess the client for signs of anxiety and embarrassment, and plan the procedure to minimize embarrassment and provide support and education. If the client is having difficulty complying, obtain a specimen later, if possible. Plan ahead, if possible, and encourage fluids before it is time to collect the specimen. Do not stand over the client, and do not stand immediately outside the door unless there is a risk of fainting or falling. If the client is embarrassed, leave the room after the explanation. Inform the client that you are leaving, and when you will return. Point out the assistance call button prior to leaving. Instruct the client to call when the specimen is collected. Use techniques to encourage urination, such as running water, applying a moist compress over the abdomen or labia in women, pouring water over the labia, and placing hands under warm water.

▶ VARIATIONS

Geriatric Variations:
- *Elderly clients may have difficulty controlling stream and need assistance in cleaning and catching the urine midstream.*
- *If arthritis is present, the client may have difficulty holding labia apart.*
- *Labia are enlarged with age and can be difficult to keep separated.*

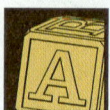

Pediatric Variations:
- *Explain the procedure to a family member.*
- *In young children parents may prefer to obtain the specimen.*
- *Teenagers may be especially embarrassed by the request for a specimen, and need control and privacy over the procedure when possible.*

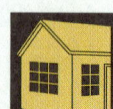

Home Care Variations:
- *Ensure that client understands the need for the sterile specimen.*
- *Specimens must be fresh and transported to the laboratory shortly after collection. Plan a specimen collection time, and a time when the specimen will be delivered to the laboratory.*
- *If specimens will be collected at home, ensure that the client has a sterile specimen cup and towelettes. Instruct clients to place container in a Ziploc® bag and refrigerate until it is delivered to a laboratory; this prevents the growth of bacteria and promotes accuracy of results.*

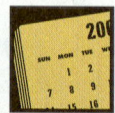

Long-Term-Care Variations:
- *Ensure that client understands the need for the sterile specimen.*
- *Specimens must be fresh and transported to the laboratory shortly after collection. Plan a specimen collection time, and a time when the specimen will be delivered to the laboratory.*
- *If specimens will be collected at home, ensure that the client has a sterile specimen cup and towelettes. Instruct clients to place container in a Ziploc® bag and refrigerate until it is delivered to a laboratory; this prevents the growth of bacteria and promotes accuracy of results.*

SKILL 1-10 Collecting a Clean-Catch, Midstream Urine Specimen

▶ COMMON ERRORS

Possible Error:
Specimen is contaminated because the client does not understand the cleaning procedure and need for the specimen to be collected midstream.

Prevention:
Explain to the client the importance of obtaining a clean specimen and the correct procedure. Ask the client to provide another sample.

Possible Error:
Specimen contaminated by labia not held apart during voiding.

Prevention:
Explain to the client the importance of obtaining a clean specimen and the correct procedure. Ask the client to provide another sample.

Possible Error:
The specimen container lid is placed upside down on a surface and contaminated.

Prevention:
Do not use the contaminated lid. Obtain a new one instead.

Possible Error:
The specimen is not labeled.

Prevention:
Always label the specimen immediately after it is obtained. There is no other way to identify the specimen.

▶ NURSING TIPS

- Labia may be slippery after cleansing; therefore, use sterile dry gauze to hold apart during urination.
- Clients often do not understand the need to remove the specimen container before completing urination; therefore, carefully explain the purpose for midstream collection.
- Encourage fluids before collecting specimen, if not contraindicated.
- If the client is unable to void, run tap water within hearing distance or place a warm compress over the bladder.
- Place the lid on a firm surface within close reach.
- Send the specimen to the laboratory immediately. It must be fresh for accurate analysis.
- Label the time of collection on the specimen.
- If a container touches the client's skin and is contaminated, obtain a new specimen cup. If necessary, arrange to have the client return to obtain another specimen.

▶ SPECIAL CONSIDERATIONS

- *Urine samples should be sent to the laboratory within 30 minutes. If this is not possible, the specimen may be refrigerated for 2–4 hours. Delaying the lab testing may alter the test results.*
- *Menstrual blood may alter the test results. In a menstruating client, perineal care should be performed before urine specimen collection, and a tampon or 4 × 4 gauze pad may be placed in the vaginal orifice to prevent contamination of urine by vaginal secretion or blood. Notify the lab of the possible presence of menstrual blood.*
- *When initiating a 24-hours urine sample, the client must void prior to starting the collection process to provide an accurate measurement.*
- *Clients with urinary tract infections may have difficulty controlling stream and need assistance.*

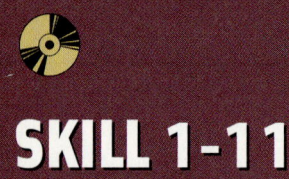

SKILL 1-11

Testing Urine for Specific Gravity, Ketones, Glucose, and Occult Blood

KEY TERMS

Gaylene Bouska Altman, RN, PhD

Diastix
Dipstick
Glucose
Ketones
Occult blood
Specific gravity
Test tape
Urine refractometer
Urinometer

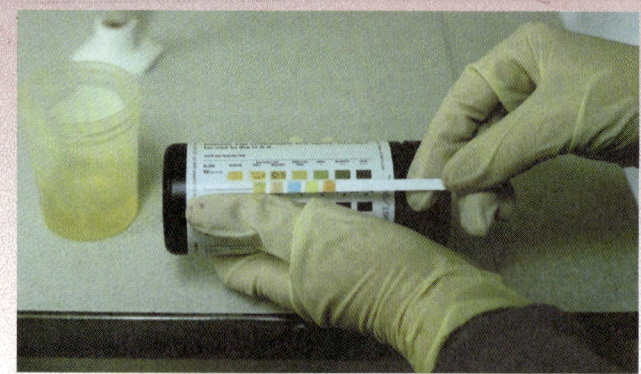

▶ **OVERVIEW OF THE SKILL**

Urine samples can be used to test specific gravity, ketones, glucose blood, pH, protein, nitrates, and bilirubin. Specific gravity is the concentration of dissolved substances in the urine compared with water. The normal range of specific gravity is between approximately 1.010 and 1.025 g/mL. If urine is dilute and less concentrated, the specific gravity will be closer to that of water with no substances, 1.000. Overhydration, or any disease that affects the ability of the body to concentrate substances in the urine, will cause a low specific gravity. Any condition that increases water reabsorption in the kidney will result in a high specific gravity.

Specific gravity testing takes only a few minutes. A rough screen can be done using a dipstick that measures specific gravity, such as a reagent strip. Reagent strips measure specific gravity through color changes, which are compared with a chart provided by the manufacturer. For greater precision, a urinometer or refractometer may be used. A urinometer measures specific gravity by displacement. Dissolved substances in the urine will push, or displace, the bulb upward. A reading is taken at the meniscus. The measurement revealed by the urinometer is a comparison of where the bulb would be floating in pure water. Concentrated particles in the urine push the bulb higher and yield a higher reading. A refractometer measures specific gravity using the refraction of light as it passes through a drop of urine on glass. A beam of light passing through the urine will bend and change direction. The amount of the bend, or refraction, is changed by the amount of dissolved substances in the urine. When frequent, exact measurements of specific gravity are required, refractometers are the best choice; however, refractometers are expensive compared with urinometers or dipsticks.

Test strips or dipsticks that are specific for ketones, glucose, blood, pH, proteins, nitrates, and bilirubin can be used to measure specific substances. These products use various names. Some examples and substances measured are ketostix (ketones), ketodiastix (glucose, ketones), clinistix and diastix (glucose), hemastix (blood), hemacombistix (pH, protein, glucose, blood), uristix (protein, glucose, nitrite, leukocytes), and labstix (pH, protein, glucose, ketone, blood). Many other examples are available. Other products can also be used to measure bilirubin, phenylketones, and leukocytes.

Multistix can be used to measure many possible substances (glucose, ketones, specific gravity, blood, pH, protein, nitrite, leukocytes, urobilinogen, and bilirubin). Sticks that measure multiple substances are generally more expensive. Tablets are available to measure glucose; however, these products are rarely used because dipsticks are readily available and easy to use. Many different systemic changes can cause glucose, ketones, or blood in the urine. The presence of glucose usually indicates an elevated blood glucose level (usually above 180 mg/dl); however, renal threshold can vary with each client. Most often blood glucose levels are used rather than urine glucose levels; however, this does require a venipuncture or finger prick. Ketones are present in the urine in cases of starvation, dehydration, and diabetic acidosis. The presence of ketones in the urine indicates that the body is burning fats for energy. Ketones alter the pH of urine to acidic. Blood in the urine indicates bleeding in the renal system or erythrocyte breakdown elsewhere in the body, such as in trauma. Local bleeding, such as menstruation, surgery, or a recent delivery of a baby, may cause blood in the urine.

▶ ASSESSMENT

1. Assess the client's understanding of the urine test to be performed. **Determines what education should be provided.**
2. Assess the client's hydration, such as skin turgor, condition of the mucous membranes, fontanels (in infants), sunken eyes, intake, and output. **Provides information to help determine physical status in addition to urine tests.**
3. Assess the client's history for renal function (e.g., medical history and lab values, creatinine clearance). **Influences how the results of tests might be interpreted. Influences what tests might be performed.**
4. If measuring glucose, assess the client for signs and symptoms of increased glucose (polyuria, polydypsia, polyphagia, recent loss of weight, fatigue). **Provides information to help determine physical status in addition to urine tests.**
5. If the client is to perform long-term tests, assess the client's ability to perform the tests. **Determines what education should be provided.**

▶ DIAGNOSIS

- Excess Fluid Volume.
- Deficient Fluid Volume.
- Imbalanced Nutrition: More than Body Requirements.
- Imbalanced Nutrition: Less than Body Requirements.
- Deficient Knowledge Regarding Urine Testing (e.g., client with elevated glucose).

▶ PLANNING

Expected Outcomes:

1. Normal specific gravity.
2. Absence of glucose and ketones in the urine.

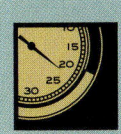

Estimated time to complete the skill:
5 minutes to collect urine;
5 minutes to perform test

3. The client understands the purpose of the test.
4. The client understands how to perform the test (if it is needed on a long-term basis).

Equipment Needed (see Figure 1-11-1):

- Urine specimen container
- Urinometer or refractometer for specific gravity
- Dipstick specific to product to measure
- Nonsterile gloves
- Watch or clock

▶ CLIENT EDUCATION NEEDED

1. Carefully explain the purpose of the test.
2. Instruct the client on the need for an uncontaminated specimen.
3. Instruct the client on the need for a second voided specimen for accuracy.
4. If the test is abnormal, explain what changes are necessary, e.g., increased glucose or dietary changes.

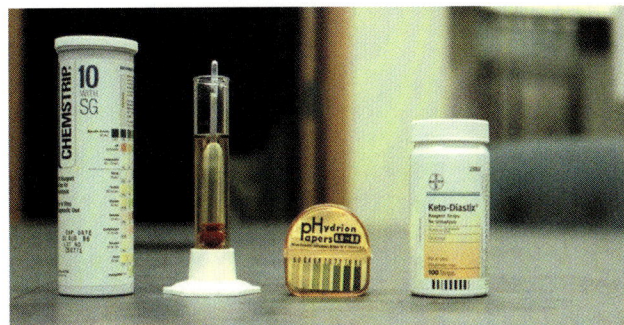

Figure 1-11-1 Reagent strips, pH papers, and urinometers are used to test urine for concentration, pH level, and specific substances, such as blood or ketones.

▶ DELEGATION TIP

Testing urine is routinely delegated to properly trained ancillary personnel. The prompt reporting of abnormal results and the recording of all results on the correct clinical records are essential.

IMPLEMENTATION—ACTION/RATIONALE

ACTION	RATIONALE
Overview—Measuring Specific Gravity	
1. Wash hands. Apply nonsterile gloves.	1. Reduces the transmission of microorganisms.
2. Obtain urine from the client either via clean-catch method (Chapter 1, Skill 1-10) or from catheter.	2. Acquires a pure sample for testing.
3. Measure the specific gravity using equipment available in your facility.	3. Obtains a measurement using equipment available in your facility.
4. Discard urine according to standard precautions.	4. Reduces the transmission of microorganisms.
5. Remove gloves and wash hands.	5. Reduces the transmission of microorganisms.
6. Clean the equipment with soap and water or according to the manufacturer's instructions.	6. Reduces the transmission of microorganisms, and prepares equipment for the next use.
7. Record the results and compare with the previous recording.	7. Allow for accuracy and monitoring of the client.
Using a Digital Clinical Refractometer to Measure Specific Gravity	
8. To use a digital refractometer (see Figure 1-11-2), become familiar with the manufacturer's instructions.	8. Ensures an accurate test.
9. Use an eye dropper to drip urine onto the prism at the center of the stainless steel stage until the prism is covered.	9. Following the manufacturer's instructions ensures an accurate reading.

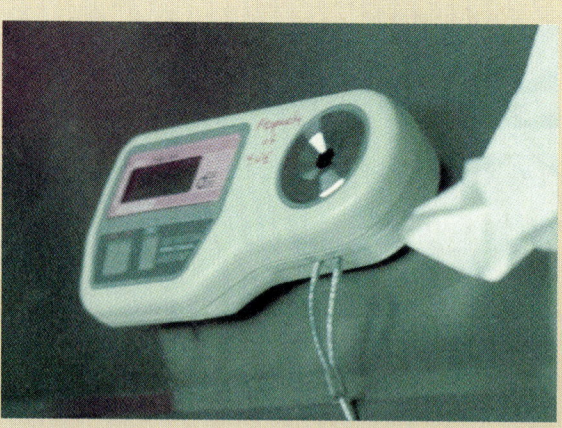

Figure 1-11-2 Digital refractometer is to measure urine specific gravity.

SKILL 1-11 Testing Urine for Specific Gravity, Ketones, Glucose, and Occult Blood

10. Press the start/off button, or the button designated by the manufacturer, to activate the meter. The specific gravity reading is displayed.

10. Following the manufacturer's instructions ensures an accurate reading.

Using a Nondigital Refractometer to Measure Specific Gravity

11. For a urine refractometer: Collect a few drops of urine.

11. Refractometers require only a drop or two of urine to measure specific gravity.

12. Place a drop of urine on the horizontal glass slide at the top of the scope.

12. Following the manufacturer's instructions ensures an accurate reading.

13. Close the cover over the slide and turn on the light.

13. Following the manufacturer's instructions ensures an accurate reading.

14. Look through the scope with one eye while keeping both eyes open.

14. It is easier to visualize if both eyes are kept open.

15. Read the number at the line where the top black and lower white circles meet. Write down the number.

15. Following the manufacturer's instructions ensures an accurate reading. Records an accurate reading because refractors are often kept in the utility room away from charting area.

16. Clean the slide with a damp towel or gauze, or according to manufacturer's recommendations.

16. Ensures equipment is ready for next use.

Using a Urinometer to Measure Specific Gravity

17. To measure specific gravity with a urinometer, at least 20 cc of urine are needed. Pour fresh urine specimen into glass cylinder to indicated line of urinometer, approximately 2/3 to 3/4 full (see Figure 1-11-3).

17. There must be enough time to make the bulb float, but it should not overfill the urinometer. The bulb should not touch the bottom of the urinometer. The meniscus of urine should be slightly below the top of the urinometer.

18. Place urinometer on flat surface and gently spin the top of the glass stem (see Figure 1-11-4).

18. Necessary to obtain an accurate reading.

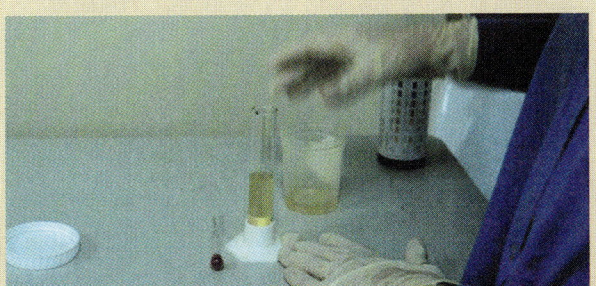

Figure 1-11-3 Fill the glass cylinder to the line with fresh urine.

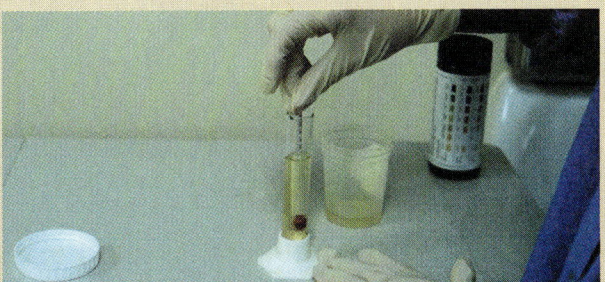

Figure 1-11-4 Spin the glass stem in the urine.

continues

Using a Urinometer to Measure Specific Gravity continued

19. Wait until the stem stops moving up and down, then visualize the urinometer scale at eye level. Read at lowest point of meniscus where the urine level touches the calibrated scale (see Figure 1-11-5).

19. Necessary to obtain accurate results.

Using a Dipstick to Test Urine for Glucose, Ketones, Occult Blood, or Specific Gravity

20. Collect a clean voided specimen.

20. Ensures accurate results.

21. Obtain the correct product for testing. Check the expiration date.

21. Products vary according to what is being measured. An expired product may produce an inaccurate reading.

22. Review the instructions on the label. Visualize which color scale will be used.

22. Accurate timing of reading is necessary for accurate results. Different manufacturers and different products require different procedures.

23. Follow the directions. The dipstick will usually be dipped into the container of urine and read at a specified time interval and according to a color scale on the bottle or tape holder, as indicated by the manufacturer's instructions (see Figure 1-11-6).

23. Direction may vary according to the product used. Check manufacturer's accompanying instructions for color indicator scale and time to be read.

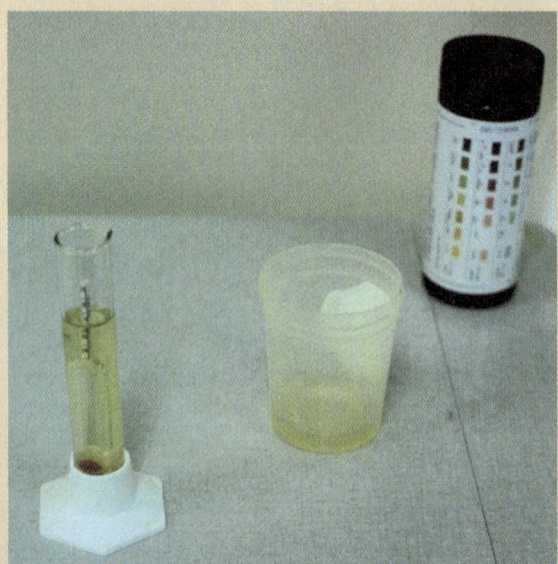

Figure 1-11-5 Read the calibrated scale when the stem stops spinning.

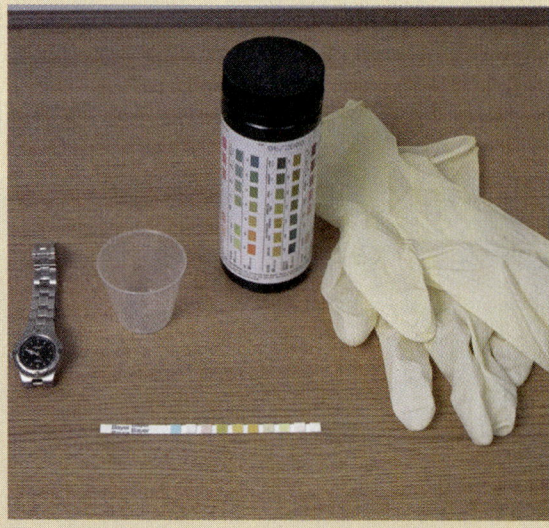

Figure 1-11-6 After dipping in fresh urine, wait the specified time interval before interpreting the results.

24. Record the results.	**24.** Because the procedure is generally done in the utility room, results should be written down so accurate information will be transferred to the chart.
25. Discard the urine and strip according to standard precautions.	**25.** Reduces the transmission of microorganisms.
26. Remove gloves and wash hands.	**26.** Reduces the transmission of microorganisms.

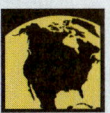

▶ **REAL WORLD ANECDOTES**

One nurse recalls her early nursing days and a particular learning curve. When she knew she needed to do a urine test using a dipstick, she would grab a strip from the bottle in the supply room and carry it down the hall to the client's room. She would then dip it in the sample in the client's bathroom and subsequently realize that she needed to compare it to the chart on the container that was sitting down the hall in the supply room.

▶ **EVALUATION**

- Evaluate the test results, and compare them with the previous results.
- Evaluate the color of the urine and any abnormal changes.

▶ **DOCUMENTATION**

Nurses' Notes

- Document the procedure and results.
- Document any visual changes noted in the urine.

▶ **CRITICAL THINKING SKILL**

Introduction

Nurses should be able to evaluate visual changes in urine and the results of the test.

Possible Scenario

Your client comes in for a routine outpatient visit and physical exam. You need a urine sample, so you instruct the client on the procedure for obtaining a clean-catch urine specimen. The client returns from the bathroom with the specimen, which looks dark. You perform the test for occult blood, and the result is positive.

Possible Outcome

You question the client further and discover that prior to voiding she removed her tampon so that the string would not dangle in the cup. You determine that the urine has been contaminated with blood from menstruation. You make arrangements to have the client return later in the afternoon to provide a second specimen.

Prevention

Since you cannot cover every possible contingency when providing instruction on how to collect a clean-catch urine sample, teach the client the importance of the goal to obtain uncontaminated urine for accurate testing.

▶ VARIATIONS

Geriatric Variations:
- Elderly clients may have a more difficult time collecting uncontaminated urine. Women especially may have difficulty because of labial changes that occur with age. They may need more careful assistance or instruction in collecting specimens.
- Elderly clients may have a difficult time reading the small print on the label or the color scale and may need assistance or a magnifying glass.

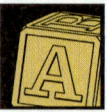
Pediatric Variations:
- A specific gravity can be obtained with a urine refractometer even with only a drop or two of urine from a wet diaper.
- Normal specific gravity values may vary slightly for children.

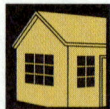
Home Care Variation:
- Contamination of the specimen may occur. Carefully instruct the client on the need for a clean-catch and second-voided specimen.

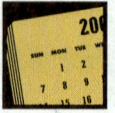
Long-Term-Care Variation:
- Instruct the client and caregiver on the need to use dipsticks or test tapes that are not past the expiration date. To save money, some clients may cut test tapes; doing so increases the risk for inaccurate readings.

▶ COMMON ERRORS

Possible Error:
Overfilling the urinometer with urine.

Prevention:
Avoid pouring from a large container with a large volume of urine. It is more difficult to control. Note carefully how much urine is needed to fill the urinometer to the correct amount.

Possible Error:
Urine contaminated with feces.

Prevention:
Remind the client that the urine is being measured and tested when you place the bedpan, commode, or escort the client to the bathroom.

Possible Error:
Inaccurate timing with test strip if instructions not read ahead of time.

Prevention:
Read the instructions before testing the urine.

SKILL 1-11 Testing Urine for Specific Gravity, Ketones, Glucose, and Occult Blood

▶ NURSING TIPS

- Visualize urine before tests to look for contamination.
- Read instructions before dipping stick or test tape in urine.
- Have at least 20 cc of urine for urinometer.
- Verify that the urine is a second-voided specimen and explain this need to the client.

▶ SPECIAL CONSIDERATIONS

- *Normally, ketones, blood, glucose and protein are absent in the urine. However, consuming a high-carbohydrate meal may result in glucosuria. In female clients, blood may be present in the urine during menstruation. Blood may be present in the urine of clients on anticoagulants or high doses of aspirin.*
- *Conditions such as strenuous exercise and starvation that increase the fatty acid metabolism can cause ketoacidosis, resulting in ketone bodies in the urine.*
- *Secretions from the penis or vagina can cause false readings of proteinuria. Obtaining a thorough health history and a clean specimen is important for the diagnostic purpose.*

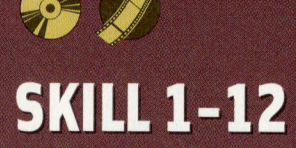

SKILL 1-12
Performing a Skin Puncture

Karrin Johnson, RN and Gaylene Bouska Altman, RN, PhD

KEY TERMS

Capillary
Edematous
Lancet
Microhematocrit
Micropipette

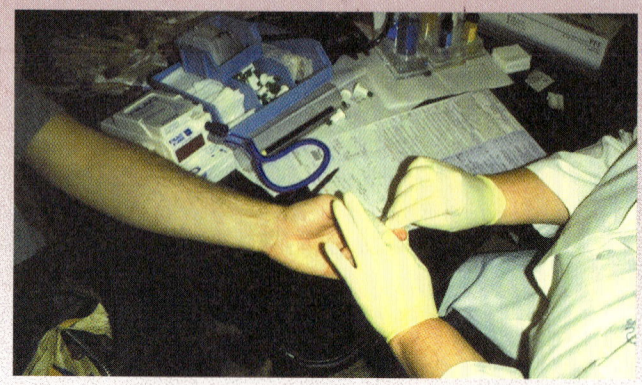

▶ OVERVIEW OF THE SKILL

Skin punctures are performed when small quantities of capillary blood are needed for analysis or when the client has poor veins. Capillary puncture is also commonly performed for blood glucose analysis. The common sites for capillary punctures follow:

- Heel—most common site for neonates and infants
- Fingertip—the inner aspect of palmar fingertip used most commonly in children and adults
- Earlobe—used when the client is in shock or the extremities are edematous

▶ ASSESSMENT

1. Assess the condition of the client's skin at the potential puncture site **to determine if it is intact, free of bruising, and can be used without causing undue trauma to the site.**
2. Assess the circulation at the potential puncture site **to determine if it is a good site to obtain a sample, and to determine if healing at the site might be compromised.**
3. Assess the client's comfort level regarding the procedure **to determine client education and support needed.**
4. Assess the cleanliness of the client's skin **to determine how much cleansing is needed prior to the skin puncture.**

▶ DIAGNOSIS

- Risk for Impaired Skin Integrity.
- Pain.
- Anxiety.

▶ PLANNING

Expected Outcomes:

1. An adequate blood specimen will be obtained.
2. The client will suffer minimal trauma during the specimen collection.
3. The specimen will be collected and stored in a manner compatible with the ordered tests.

Equipment Needed (see Figure 1-12-1):

- Antiseptic 70% isopropanol or povidone-iodine
- Microhematocrit tubes or micropipette (collection tubes)
- Sterile 2 × 2 gauze
- Sterile lancet
- Nonsterile gloves
- Hand towel or absorbent pad

▶ CLIENT EDUCATION NEEDED

1. Explain the reason that the lateral aspect of the finger is used to avoid the nerve endings at the tip of the finger.

SKILL 1-12 Performing a Skin Puncture

2. Inform the client that a small sharp prick will occur.
3. Tell the client to hold pressure on the site for several minutes following the blood collection to prevent seepage of blood into the tissues.

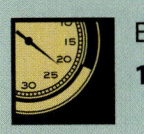
Estimated time to complete the skill: **15 minutes**

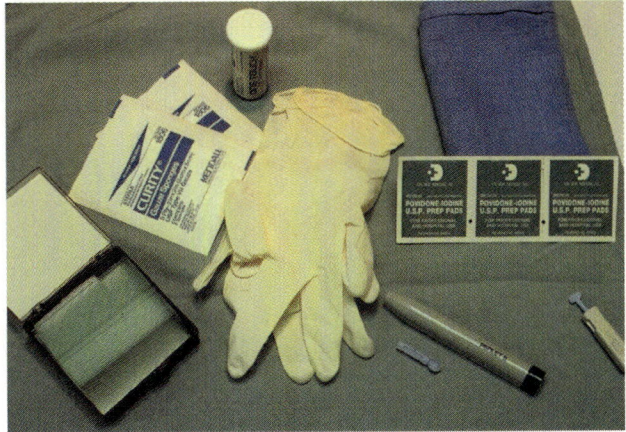
Figure 1-12-1 Various lancet devices, alcohol wipes, povidone-iodine, gauze, and gloves.

▶ DELEGATION TIPS

Properly trained ancillary personnel may perform skin puncture. Agency policy usually dictates certification and recertification requirements for this skill. Proper patient and specimen identification are of the utmost importance and must be consistently demonstrated by the ancillary personnel.

IMPLEMENTATION—ACTION/RATIONALE

ACTION	RATIONALE
1. Wash hands.	1. Reduces transmission of microorganisms.
2. Check the client's identification band if appropriate.	2. Ensures the correct client.
3. Explain the procedure to the client.	3. Allays anxiety and encourages cooperation.
4. Prepare supplies: • Open sterile packages. • Label specimen collection tubes. • Place in easy reach.	4. Ensures efficiency.
5. Apply gloves.	5. Decreases the health care provider's exposure to blood-borne organisms.
6. Select site: Lateral aspect of the fingertips in adults/children. Heel for neonates and infants.	6. Avoid damage to nerve endings and calloused areas of the skin.

continues

continued

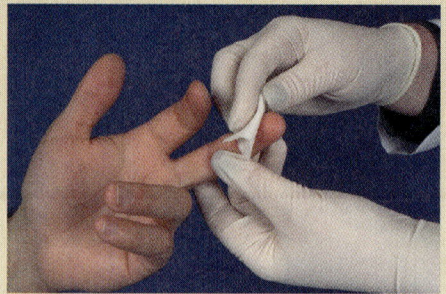

Figure 1-12-2 Cleanse the puncture site, and allow it to dry.

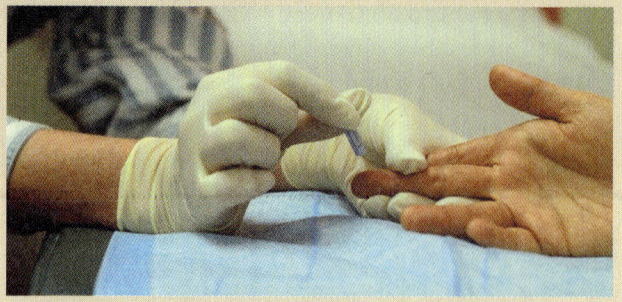

Figure 1-12-3 Use a quick stab to puncture the skin.

7. Place the hand or heel in a dependent position; apply warm compresses if fingers or heel is cool to touch.

8. Place hand towel or absorbent pad under the extremity.

9. Cleanse puncture site with an antiseptic, and allow to dry. Use 70% isopropanol if the client is allergic to iodine (see Figure 1-12-2).

10. With nondominant hand, apply gentle milking pressure above or around the puncture site. Do not touch the puncture site.

11. Read directions carefully before using the lancet.
    - With the sterile lancet at a 90-degree angle to the skin, use a quick stab to puncture the skin (about 2 mm deep) (see Figure 1-12-3).
    - With the automatic unistik, push the lancet into the body of unistik until it clicks. Hold the body of the unistik and twist off the lancet cap. Place the end of the unistik tightly against the client's finger and press the lever. The needle automatically retracts after use.

12. Wipe off the first drop of blood with sterile 2 × 2 gauze; allow the blood to flow freely (see Figure 1-12-4).

13. Collect the blood into the tube(s). If blood for a platelet count is to be collected, obtain this specimen first (see Figure 1-12-5).

7. Increases the blood supply to the puncture site.

8. Prevents soiling the bed linen.

9. Reduces skin surface bacteria; povidone-iodine must dry to be effective.

10. Increases blood to puncture site and maintains asepsis.

11. Provides a blood sample with minimal discomfort to the client.

12. The first drop may contain a large amount of serous fluid, which could affect the results. Pressure at the puncture site can cause hemolysis.

13. Allows blood collection; avoids aggregation of platelets at the puncture site.

SKILL 1-12 Performing a Skin Puncture

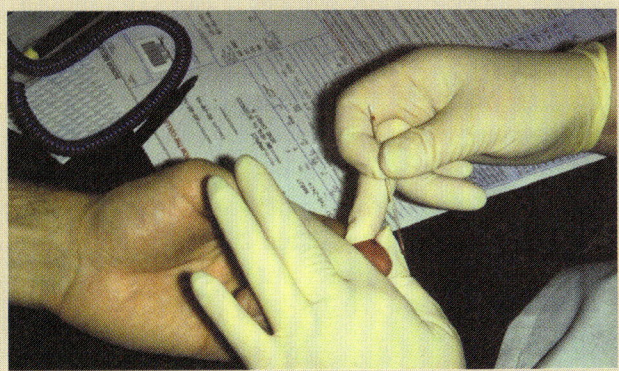

Figure 1-12-4 Allow the blood to flow from the puncture site to ensure an adequate amount can be obtained.

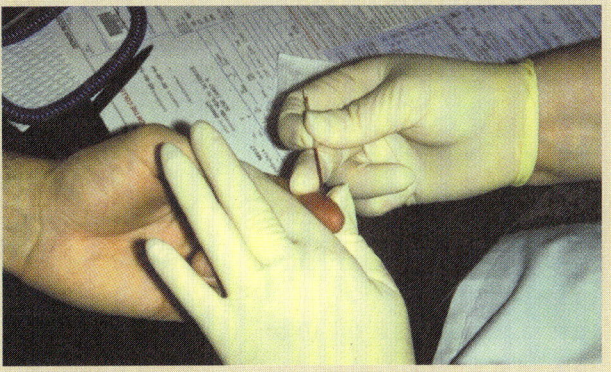

Figure 1-12-5 Collect a small sample of blood.

14. Apply pressure to the puncture site with a sterile 2 × 2 gauze (see Figure 1-12-6).

15. Place contaminated articles into a sharps container.

16. Remove gloves; wash hands.

17. Position client for comfort with call light in reach.

18. Wash hands.

14. Controls bleeding.

15. Reduces the risk of needle stick.

16. Reduces transmission of microorganisms.

17. Provides for comfort and communication.

18. Reduces transmission of microorganisms.

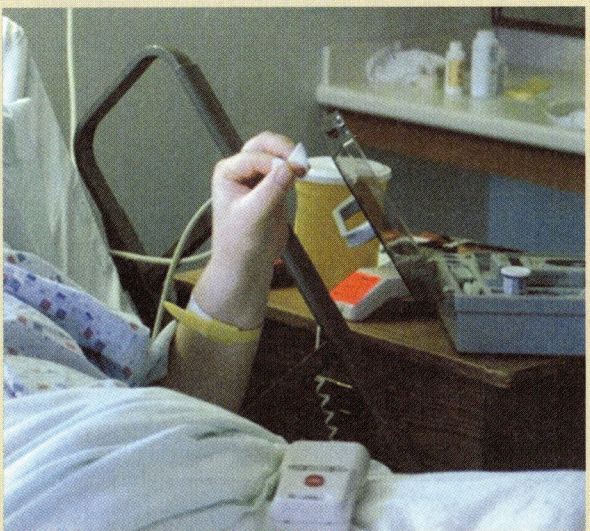

Figure 1-12-6 Apply pressure to the puncture site to stop further bleeding.

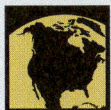

▶ REAL WORLD ANECDOTES

While performing capillary puncture for blood glucose monitoring, the nurse noted that despite what appeared to be an adequate puncture, the site was not bleeding. In an attempt to encourage a free flow of blood, the nurse gently squeezed the client's fingertip. Blood suddenly squirted from the puncture site, spraying the nurse's face. It is a good idea not to squeeze the area of a skin puncture but to let the blood flow freely.

▶ EVALUATION

- Determine that the specimen is adequate.
- Evaluate the client's condition for trauma.

▶ DOCUMENTATION

Nurses' Notes

- Document the puncture site and the reason for the puncture.
- Report test results if the testing is performed at the time of the puncture.

▶ CRITICAL THINKING SKILL

Introduction

It is important to put the client at ease as much as possible.

Possible Scenario

A local company is offering free cholesterol tests. The sample is obtained using skin puncture and a capillary tube. Because of an unexpectedly large turnout at lunchtime, some clients have been waiting in line for an hour. A heavy-set male client sits down to have his cholesterol tested. He is pale and diaphoretic. He notes that he has always been frightened of any kind of needles and has fainted in the past. His stomach is growling.

Possible Outcome

The nurse feels pressure to work quickly because of the long line. She ignores the client's words and fails to note his physical symptoms. As she begins, the client complains of "feeling queasy," then abruptly tumbles from the chair in a faint. Supplies and tubes tumble with him, and the chair is knocked over. The waiting line shortens considerably.

Prevention

Skin puncture is a frightening procedure to most people. Many people have unpleasant memories regarding this procedure. This client's apprehension regarding the procedure caused him to faint. Prior to performing a skin puncture to obtain a capillary sample, the nurse should have allowed the client to sit a few minutes and talk about his concerns regarding the procedure. He needed to be reassured that skin puncture is done with a much smaller and sharper blade than in the past. If the client continued to seem pale and perhaps hypoglycemic, the nurse should have encouraged him to go eat lunch and come back a little later. Only perform the test if the client's condition seems stable. Be prepared if the client faints or vomits.

▶ VARIATIONS

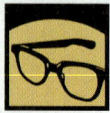

Geriatric Variation:
- *The elderly often have very thin, fragile skin. When performing capillary puncture, be careful not to tear the skin.*

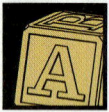

Pediatric Variation:
- *The heel is the most frequently used site for infants and neonates. Placing a warm pack on the infant's heel often increases the blood flow from the puncture site.*

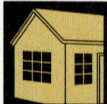

Home Care Variations:
- *The home care client should be encouraged to rotate sites even if this is awkward at first.*
- *Teach the home care client to maintain sharp lancets for capillary puncture by frequently changing lancets rather than using the same one repeatedly.*

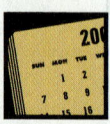

Long-Term-Care Variation:
- *Clients who require frequent capillary puncture for blood level monitoring should be encouraged to rotate the sites used for puncture. Using both lateral aspects of all fingers can help prevent soreness and bruising at any one site.*

▶ COMMON ERRORS

Possible Error:

The puncture is too shallow to obtain a sufficient specimen.

Prevention:

This problem is usually resolved with practice. Think to yourself, why wasn't the puncture deep enough to obtain enough blood? Could this be the result of poor equipment or poor technique? Is the puncture blade sharp enough? Is the lancet designed to enter skin to a measured depth and then retract? Did I use enough force to puncture the skin deeply enough? There are a number of devices on the market designed specifically for skin puncture. Try several types of devices until you find one you are comfortable using. Occasionally, the blade is not pressed tightly enough against the skin to obtain a deep, clean puncture. Be sure to use enough force to hold the puncture device tightly enough against the skin to obtain a deep, clean puncture.

▶ NURSING TIPS

- Have the client hold his hand in a dependent position while you are setting up the equipment to promote venous engorgement in the fingertips.
- Be sure the client's hands are warm.
- Use the client's nondominant hand, if possible.

▶ SPECIAL CONSIDERATIONS

- *The puncture site may be cleaned with warm, soapy water instead of an alcohol swab. Constant alcohol prepping may result in thickening of the skin and make future fingersticks more painful. The warmth of the water helps to increase peripheral blood circulation.*
- *A less painful procedure can be achieved by choosing the sides of fingertips, which have fewer nerve endings compared with the soft, central part of the fingertips.*
- *A stroking or milking technique toward the fingertip can facilitate obtaining a maximum amount of blood.*

SKILL 1-13

Measuring Blood Glucose Levels

Susan Weiss Behrend, RN, PhD, Catherine H. Kelley, RN, MSN, OCN, and Susan Randolph, RN, MSN, CS

KEY TERMS

Blood glucose meters
Blood glucose monitoring
Blood glucose testing
Capillary blood glucose
Diabetes management
Insulin management

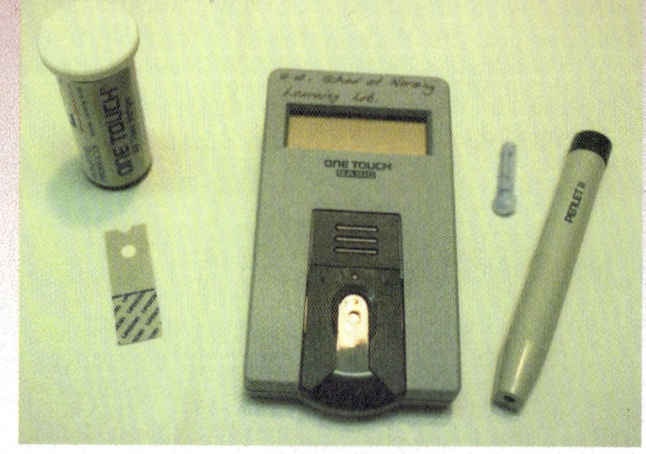

▸ OVERVIEW OF THE SKILL

Advances in technology have enabled the nurse, client, and/or caregiver to perform some laboratory tests at the bedside or in the home setting. Blood glucose monitoring, using either reagent strips or glucose meters, combined with a skin puncture lancet, is an example of such technology. The convenience of this test has dramatically changed the ongoing management of many clients, particularly those with diabetes.

Testing of blood glucose can be done by obtaining a blood sample through venipuncture or by obtaining capillary blood with a skin puncture. In situations requiring frequent blood glucose monitoring, the preferred method of blood sampling is the skin puncture technique.

There are primarily two methods used to measure blood glucose. Both methods require a large drop of blood obtained through skin puncture with a sterile lancet. The first method requires that the drop of blood be applied to a special chemical reagent strip. The participant visually compares the reagent strip to a color chart on the reagent container. Accuracy may be compromised if the result falls between two colors and the participant must estimate the blood glucose level. Examples of reagent strips include Chemstrip BG, Glucostix, and Trendstrips.

A second method of blood glucose monitoring replaces the visual comparison method with the use of a portable meter. Once the blood is placed on the reagent strip, the meter provides an accurate measurement of the blood glucose. There are a variety of meters available, including Accu-Check Advantage (Accu-Check), Accu-Check Active (Accu-Check), Bayer Elite (Bayer), Glucometer (Bayer), One Touch II (Lifescan), Sure Step Pro (Lifescan), InDuo (Lifescan), and Precision (Medisense). Because models vary and technology continues to evolve, it is essential that the nurse or client using the device review the specific manufacturer's operating guidelines and be familiar with the equipment. Failure to do so could compromise the test results.

▸ ASSESSMENT

1. Review the physician's or qualified practitioner's order for glucose monitoring **to determine if the order specifies the method (reagent strip versus meter).**
2. Identify which type of equipment is available at your facility. **It is imperative to be knowledgeable of the type of method used and specific meter that is available for use. Accurate tests results depend on proper use of all equipment involved.**
3. Review the client's medical history for diabetes, visual impairment, or anticoagulant therapy. **A thorough knowledge of the client's medical history is**

important—even when the test performed is a relatively simple procedure. Visual impairment or other disabilities can hinder self-care and may affect test results. Anticoagulant therapy may result in prolonged bleeding at the skin puncture site and require pressure to the site.

4. Determine if the test requires special timing, e.g., before or after meals. **Blood glucose levels are affected by diet, and the test may be scheduled at very specific intervals. Therapy orders are based on the assumption that the test results are accurate.**
5. Assess the client's or caregiver's ability to manage the equipment and perform the test accurately if the care will be provided at home. **Proper client/caregiver education is essential; clients/caregivers should return demonstrate their ability to carry out the test and clean the equipment before they assume such a responsibility.**
6. Assess the client's understanding of the rationale for the test and the importance of accurate results. Determine the client's willingness to perform the test, and identify if the client will incorporate the test schedule into daily routine. **Compliance with the expected schedule and procedure is more likely to occur when the client is knowledgeable about the rationale for the procedure. Some clients may have difficulty with some aspects of the procedure, such as the finger stick, and may be unwilling to participate in self-care.**
7. Assess the client's sites for skin puncture. **Sites should have good skin integrity in order to minimize risk of infection and promote healing.**

▸ DIAGNOSIS

- Anxiety. The client may have anxiety or fear related to the procedure of skin puncture.
- Anxiety. The client may have anxiety related to a diagnosis of diabetes.

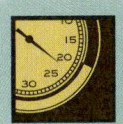

Estimated time to complete the skill: 10 minutes

- Risk for Impaired Skin Integrity. The client may have an alteration in skin integrity related to the diagnosis.
- Disturbed Sensory Perception. The client may have an alteration in visual acuity or sensorium related to the disease process.

▸ PLANNING

Expected Outcomes:

1. Blood glucose level is maintained within a normal range.
2. Client/caregiver demonstrates accurate performance of the procedure.
3. Client verbalizes an understanding of the importance of the test and the need for accurate results.
4. Client verbalizes minimal anxiety associated with the procedure.
5. Skin puncture sites remain free of signs and symptoms of infection.

Equipment Needed (see Figures 1-13-1 and 1-13-2):

- Reagent strips
- Disposable gloves
- Lancet or automatic lancing device
- Paper towels
- Alcohol wipe
- 2 × 2 gauze
- Cotton ball
- Blood glucose meter

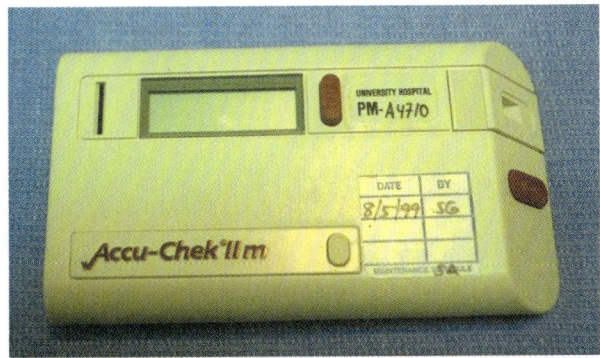

Figure 1-13-1 Blood glucose meter. There are many types and brands of glucose meters available.

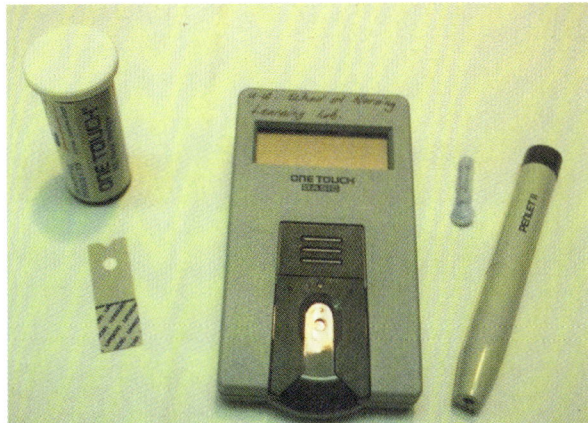

Figure 1-13-2 Test strips, blood glucose meter, and penlette.

CLIENT EDUCATION NEEDED

1. Explain the purpose and schedule for the test.
2. Provide information related to how the test results will affect the client's disease state management.
3. Discuss the time it will take for the client to master the skill.
4. When possible, include the caregiver in the teaching session to provide backup for the client in the home setting. Provide written instructions.
5. Provide information to clients regarding providers who can supply equipment needed for their diabetes care.
6. Require the learner to return demonstrate the procedure—including proper management of the equipment (cleaning, storage).
7. Help clients determine resources available if the meter malfunctions.
8. Help clients determine what their insurance plan covers related to nursing care, equipment, and medication needs.
9. Offer information on local and national organizations that provide information or support to clients with diabetes.
10. Review Standard Precautions with the client/caregiver.

DELEGATION TIPS

Properly trained ancillary personnel may measure blood glucose levels. Agency and state health department policies usually dictate certification and recertification requirements for this skill. Proper patient and specimen identification are of the utmost importance and must be consistently demonstrated by the ancillary personnel. Proper recording of results and prompt reporting to the nurse of abnormal findings are essential.

IMPLEMENTATION—ACTION/RATIONALE

ACTION	RATIONALE
1. Review orders, identify the client, and review the manufacturer's instructions for meter usage.	1. Prevents performing an invasive procedure on the wrong client, and promotes accuracy of results.
2. Wash hands.	2. Reduces transmission of microorganisms.
3. Assemble the equipment at the bedside (see Figure 1-13-3).	3. Allows for a smooth procedure.

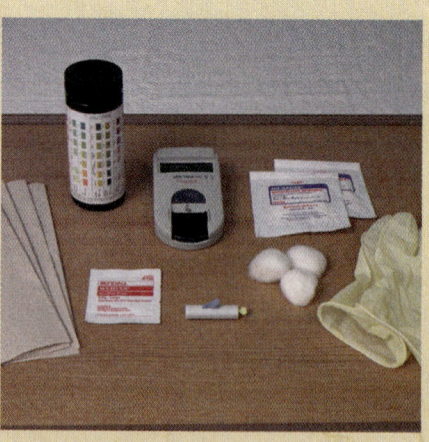

Figure 1-13-3   Supplies for blood glucose testing.

4. Have the client wash hands with soap and water, and position the client comfortably in a semi-Fowler's position or upright in a chair.

4. Reduces transmission of microorganisms, and increases blood flow to the puncture site. Avoid having the client stand during the procedure, because some clients may be prone to fainting.

5. Remove a reagent strip from the container and reseal the container cap. Then, turn on meter.

5. Tight closure of the container keeps strips from discoloring from environmental factors. Activates meter for test.

6. Following the manufacturer's instructions, calibrate the meter by inserting the strip into the meter.

6. Some meters need to be calibrated; others require the timer to be adjusted; each meter has different requirements when setting it up for use.

7. Remove the unused reagent strip from the meter and place it on a clean, dry surface (paper towel) with the test pad facing up.

7. Moisture may alter the test results.

8. Apply disposable gloves.

8. Protects from contamination by blood.

9. Select appropriate puncture site, and perform skin puncture (see Figure 1-13-4).

9. Collects blood necessary for the test.

10. Wipe away the first drop of blood from the site.

10. This drop may impede accurate results because it may contain a large amount of serous fluid.

11. Gently squeeze the site to produce a large droplet of blood.

11. Do not contaminate the site by touching it; the droplet of blood needs to be large enough to cover the test pad on the reagent strip.

12. Transfer the drop of blood to the reagent strip by carefully moving the site over the strip. The droplet should transfer without smearing (see Figure 1-13-5). (Note: Some meters require that the blood droplet be applied to the strip that is already in the meter.)

12. The test pad must absorb the droplet of blood for accurate results. Smearing of the blood will alter results.

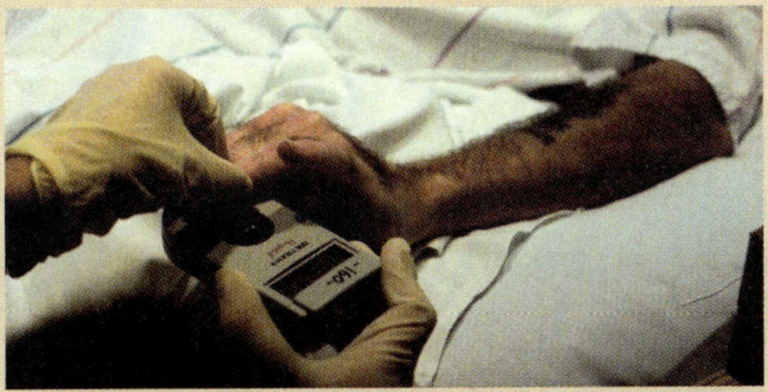

Figure 1-13-4 Perform the skin puncture.

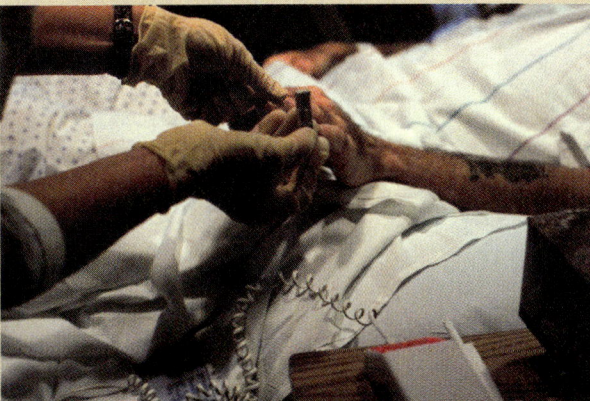

Figure 1-13-5 Transfer a drop of blood to the test strip.

continues

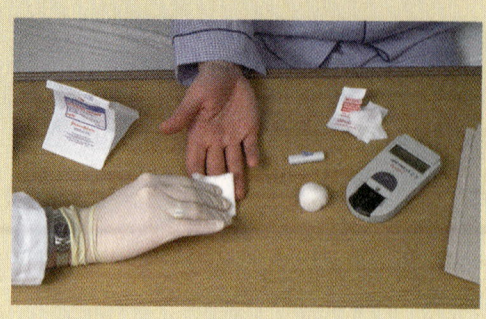

Figure 1-13-6 Apply pressure to the site.

13. Quickly press the timer on the meter and lay the strip next to the meter on a clean, dry surface.

14. Apply pressure to the puncture site (see Figure 1-13-6).

15. After 60 seconds, wipe the blood from the test pad with a cotton ball; place the strip into the meter. (Note: This step may vary with the type of meter.) Allow the timer to continue.

16. Read the meter for results found on the unit display.

17. Turn off the meter and properly dispose of the test strip, cotton ball, and lancet.

18. Remove disposable gloves, and place them in the appropriate receptacle.

19. Wash hands.

20. Review tests results with the client.

21. Notify the physician or qualified practitioner of the test results.

22. Wash hands.

13. Timing is critical to produce accurate results. Always check the manufacturer's instructions because the technique varies between meters.

14. This will stop the bleeding at the site.

15. This step is specific to certain meters (e.g., Accu-Check III) that require the strip to enter the meter dry.

16. Each meter has a specified time for the reading to occur.

17. Reduces contamination by blood to other individuals; sharps must always be handled properly to protect others from accidental injury.

18. Reduces transmission of microorganisms.

19. Reduces contamination by microorganisms.

20. Promotes participation in health care.

21. Results will be used to determine the client's treatment plan.

22. Reduces transmission of microorganisms.

▶ EVALUATION

- Reinspect the puncture site for bleeding and tissue injury.
- Compare the glucose reading to the client's previous glucose results.
- Compare the client's results to normal blood glucose levels.
- Ask the client to explain the importance of the results.
- Ask the client to return demonstrate the procedure at the next scheduled test.

▶ DOCUMENTATION

Flow Sheet

- Glucose test results
- Procedure and site used
- Appearance of puncture site

REAL WORLD ANECDOTES

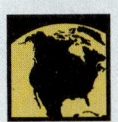

Scenario 1

Ms. Smith is an elderly woman, newly diagnosed with type 1 diabetes. The new diagnosis was overwhelming to her. She is fearful that she cannot remember all of the material that she needs to learn in order to administer insulin and test her blood glucose level. The nurse in the clinic scheduled her teaching appointments and began the process of client education. In the clinic setting, Ms. Smith gradually felt more competent with the blood glucose monitoring technique. The next day at home she tried the technique she had been taught. Her blood glucose level was significantly lower than the results she had recorded when at the clinic. She called her clinic nurse, who in turn reported the low results to the physician, who decreased her next dose of insulin. Ms. Smith was later urgently admitted for symptoms of hyperglycemia. Apparently, when reviewing information with her nurse, Ms. Smith realized she had forgotten to wipe off the first drop of blood from her finger. She had used a blood sample that was diluted with serous fluid, making her blood glucose level abnormally low. In retrospect, it would have been more appropriate to have asked Ms. Smith to recheck her results at the clinic before changing her prescription, especially because the nurse was familiar with the client's usual blood glucose levels.

Scenario 2

Kelly is a 5-year-old girl, newly diagnosed with type 1 diabetes, whose parents are becoming quite efficient in the care of their daughter. The mother demonstrated the procedure for blood glucose monitoring and felt comfortable with the procedure. However, when it was time to test Kelly's blood glucose, Kelly refused to allow her mother to puncture her finger with the lancet. After much frustration, the nurse recommended that Kelly try the automated device. With her mother's help, Kelly and her favorite doll learned how to press the release button. Eventually, as Kelly became more comfortable with the "magic button," she allowed the device to be used for her blood glucose monitoring. It is important to incorporate play into the medical care of young children and to allow them to actively participate in the process.

- Client's response to the procedure (feelings of lightheadedness, nausea, etc.)
- Abnormal results reported to physician or qualified practitioner
- Client's understanding of the procedure and ability to demonstrate the technique
- Medication Record
- Date and time insulin administered

▶ CRITICAL THINKING SKILL

Introduction

Accurate test results for blood glucose monitoring are critical because treatment decisions are based on those results. Documenting the results in a designated log/chart in the client's record is equally important.

Possible Scenario

Mr. Jones was admitted for symptoms of hyperglycemia associated with his long history of diabetes. His treatment plan included 6-hour management of his blood glucose. The nurse was very busy and neglected to document the meter reading on the flowchart. The physician asked Mr. Jones if his test had been performed. He answered "yes" and stated what meter reading he had seen on the display. The physician ordered a dose of insulin based on those results.

Possible Outcome

The obvious concern is that the meter reading was not properly documented and only anecdotal. There is considerable risk to the client if the insulin dosage is based on inaccurate blood glucose readings.

Prevention

Prompt documentation of all meter readings; notification of abnormal results to the physician or qualified practitioner; and informing the client of test results are actions that help prevent errors in this situation.

▶ VARIATIONS

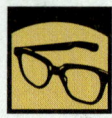

Geriatric Variations:
- *Warming fingertips will facilitate vasodilatation and collection of the blood droplet.*
- *Older clients are at risk for visual impairment; care should be taken to verify that the client is able to read the meter results accurately.*
- *Involve a caregiver in the teaching to provide backup for the elderly client, particularly in the home setting.*

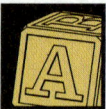

Pediatric Variations:
- *Painful procedures such as a skin puncture for a blood sample should be performed in a procedure room rather than the client's hospital room.*
- *Have assistance from staff to restrain the child or infant during the skin puncture.*
- *Topical numbing creams applied to the site prior to the puncture may reduce the discomfort associated with the test.*
- *Allow the child to choose the puncture site, when possible.*
- *Allow the child and parent to demonstrate the procedure; incorporate play activity into the procedure as needed.*
- *When using the heel of an infant, warm the foot prior to the skin puncture.*

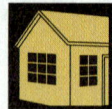

Home Care Variation:
- *Glucose monitoring meters are common devices used for home management of clients with diabetes. The nurse should note the manufacturer of the equipment and review proper maintenance and calibration of the device with the client. The nurse should also review proper disposal of equipment in the home environment.*

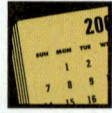

Long-Term-Care Variation:
- *In long-term-care facilities, employees performing blood glucose monitoring should be familiar with the device used for the client to ensure accurate results.*

▶ COMMON ERRORS

Possible Error:

The manufacturer's requirements were not reviewed before testing, which resulted in an inaccurate result.

Prevention:

Maintain information related to the meter in a place that is accessible to all nursing personnel. Review the specific technique required by the manufacturer.

Repeat the test using the correct technique. Select a different puncture site on the client.

▶ NURSING TIPS

- Clients admitted to the hospital who have been performing blood glucose monitoring may choose to continue to perform the procedure themselves. The nurse has an opportunity to review information, assess accuracy of the client's techniques, and offer information on new equipment that may be available.
- Clients referred to home care may rent meters from those providers. It is important that the client teaching plan is consistent with the equipment delivered to the home.
- Understand the blood glucose level "norms" for an individual client. If the new level is significantly different, suspect an error in administration of the procedure and determine other factors that may impair accurate results.

▶ SPECIAL CONSIDERATIONS

- *Avoid sharing lancet pen/holder (often supplied with glucose monitoring devices) with others, because blood-borne disease can be transmitted through lancet devices.*
- *In clients such as patients with diabetes who require regular blood glucose monitoring, "shallow penetration" should be encouraged to avoid tissue damage. Milking toward the fingertip can facilitate obtaining a maximum amount of blood. Rotate sites to allow time for the penetrated site to heal. A less painful procedure can be achieved by choosing the side of the fingertips where fewer nerve ending are located compared with the soft, central part of the fingertips.*
- *In the home health setting or in clients who perform the fingertip puncture on a regular basis, hand washing with warm, soapy water is recommended instead of using alcohol to clean the area to be punctured. Repeated cleaning of the fingerstick site with alcohol can result in thickening of the skin and make the fingerstick more painful. The warmth of the water helps increasing peripheral blood circulation.*

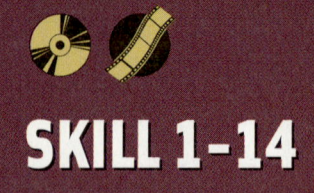

SKILL 1-14

Collecting Nose, Throat, and Sputum Specimens

Gaylene Bouska Altman, RN, PhD

KEY TERMS

Cultures
Nasal
Nasopharyngeal
Sputum
Swab
Throat

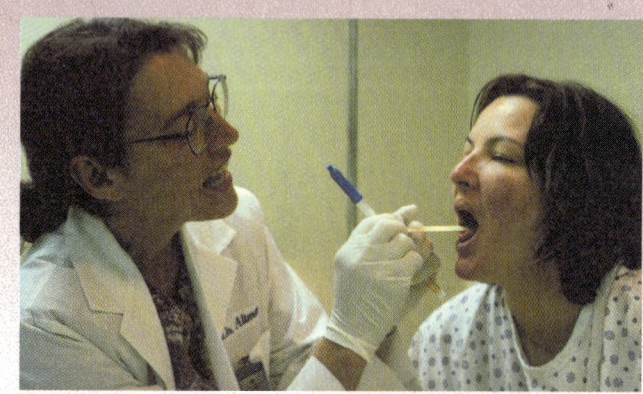

▶ OVERVIEW OF THE SKILL

A nose, throat, or sputum specimen is a simple diagnostic tool for clients with signs or symptoms of upper respiratory or sinus infections. Nose and throat specimens are collected from the client using a sterile swab. Sputum specimens are collected in a sterile cup. Sputum specimens can also be obtained via a specimen trap connected to suction. Specimens are sent to the laboratory and placed in a culture medium to allow pathogenic organisms to grow. The type of organism can be identified, enabling diagnosis and appropriate antimicrobial therapy.

▶ ASSESSMENT

1. Assess the client's understanding of the purpose of the procedure **so he will be able to cooperate.**
2. Assess the type of nasal or sinus drainage in order **to determine what kind of collection equipment will be needed.**
3. Review the physician's or qualified practitioner's orders for the cultures requested **so repeat cultures are not done.**
4. Assess the client for postnasal drip, sinus headache or tenderness, nasal congestion, or sore throat **in order to know why the procedure is being done.**
5. Identify whether the client has received recent antimicrobials and obtain a specimen prior to treatment, if possible.

▶ DIAGNOSIS

- Risk for Infection.
- Anxiety Regarding the Procedure.
- Risk for Injury.
- Deficient Knowledge Regarding the Procedure.

▶ PLANNING

Expected Outcomes:

1. An adequate specimen will be obtained and sent to the laboratory.
2. The procedure will be performed with a minimum of trauma to the client.

Equipment Needed (see Figures 1-14-1, 1-14-2, and 1-14-3):

- Two sterile swabs in sterile culture tubes or a flexible wire sterile swab with cotton tip for nose or throat cultures (see Figure 1-14-2).
- Tongue blades
- Penlight

SKILL 1-14 Collecting Nose, Throat, and Sputum Specimens

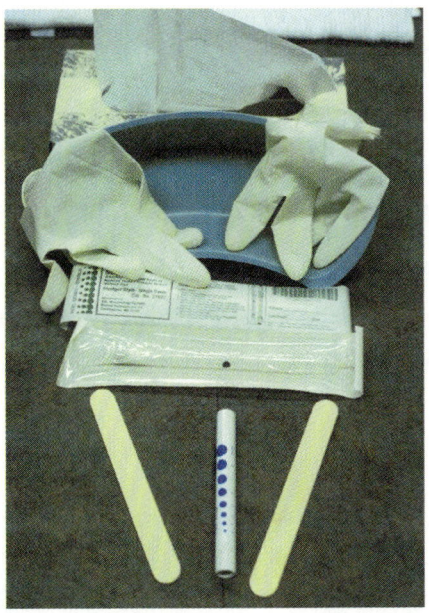

Figure 1-14-1 Penlight, tongue depressors, cotton swabs, culture medium, emesis basis, and gloves.

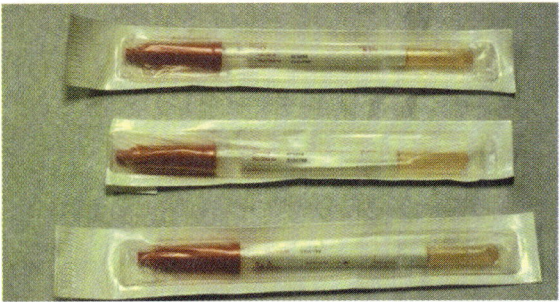

Figure 1-14-2 Prepackaged sterile swab and culture medium containers.

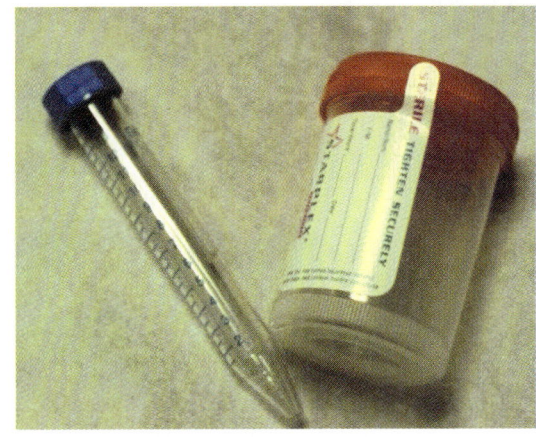

Figure 1-14-3 Sterile specimen tube and cup.

- Facial tissues
- Clean, disposable gloves
- Nasal speculum (optional)
- Emesis basin or clean container
- Sterile specimen cup, or sputum specimen collector

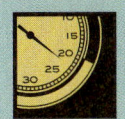 Estimated time to complete the skill: **5–10 minutes**

▶ CLIENT EDUCATION NEEDED

1. Clients should be taught the rationale for the procedure.
2. Even though the procedure is generally painless, clients should be alerted that gagging may occur.
3. Discuss the rationale for obtaining the culture.
4. Discuss the time delay for the culture results.
5. Remind the client that the culture collection requires cooperation.

▶ DELEGATION TIPS

Sputum specimens may be obtained by ancillary personnel. Avoiding specimen collection immediately after meals is important as is the use of standard precautions when handling the specimen. Obtaining nose and throat cultures requires problem-solving skills and techniques, indicating the obtaining of these specimens may not be delegated.

IMPLEMENTATION—ACTION/RATIONALE

ACTION

1. Wash hands and put on clean gloves.

2. Ask the client to sit erect in the bed or on a chair facing the nurse.

3. Prepare a sterile swab for use by loosening the top of the container (see Figure 1-14-4).

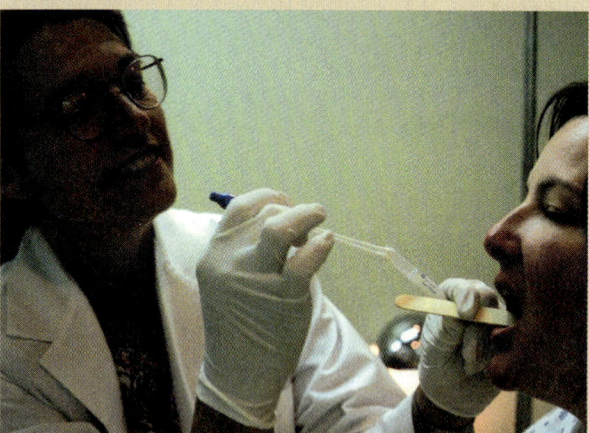

Figure 1-14-4 Loosen the swab top from container.

Collecting Throat Culture

4. Ask the client to tilt the head backward, open the mouth, and say "ah."

5. Depress the anterior one third of the tongue with a tongue blade for better visualization (see Figure 1-14-5).

6. Insert the swab without touching the cheek, lips, teeth, or tongue.

7. Swab the tonsillar area from side to side in a quick, gentle motion (see Figure 1-14-6).

8. Withdraw the swab without touching adjacent structures and place in the culture tube. Crush ampoule at bottom of tube, and push swab into liquid medium (see Figure 1-14-7).

RATIONALE

1. Reduces transmission of microorganisms.

2. Provides easy access to the nose or throat.

3. Prevents contamination of the swab.

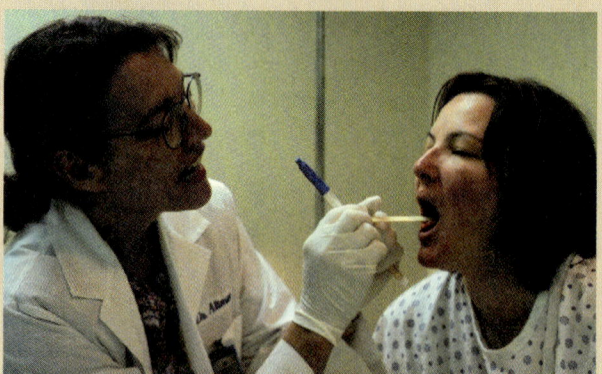

Figure 1-14-5 Depress the tongue with the tongue blade.

4. Promotes visualization of the pharynx, relaxes the throat muscles, and minimizes the gag reflex.

5. Promotes visualization of the pharynx, but may induce the gag reflex.

6. Prevents contamination of the specimen with oral flora.

7. Ensures collection of microorganisms. Retains microorganisms in the culture tube, and ensures the life of bacteria for testing.

8. Prevents contamination from outside microorganisms and erroneous culture results.

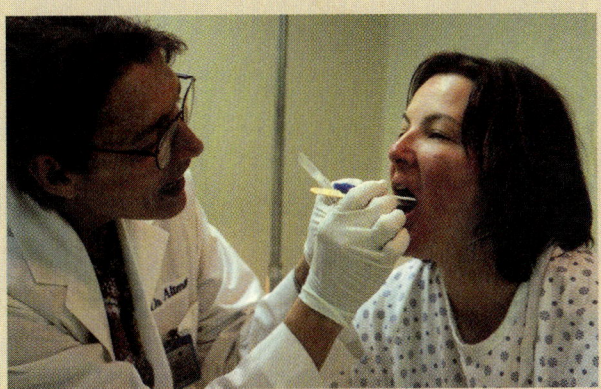

Figure 1-14-6 Swab the sample area using a quick, gentle motion.

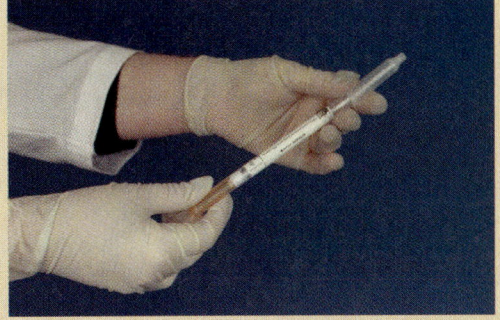

Figure 1-14-7 Crush ampoule to release the culture medium.

9. Secure the top to the culture tube and label with the client's name.

10. Discard the tongue depressor. Remove gloves and discard. Wash hands.

Collecting Nose Culture

11. Instruct the client to blow nose and check nostrils for patency with penlight.

12. Ask the client to occlude one nostril, then the other, and exhale.

13. Ask the client to tilt the head back.

14. Insert the swab into the nostril until it reaches the inflamed mucosa, and rotate the swab.

15. Withdraw the swab without touching adjacent structures and place in culture tube. Crush ampoule at bottom of tube, and push swab into liquid medium.

16. Secure the top to the culture tube and label with the client's name.

17. Remove gloves and discard. Wash hands.

Collecting of Nasopharyngeal Culture

18. Follow Actions 11–17 except use a swab on a flexible wire that can reach the nasopharynx via the nose.

9. Prevents identification mistakes.

10. Reduces transmission of microorganisms.

11. Clears nasal passages of mucus containing resident bacteria.

12. Determines the optimal nasal passage from which to obtain the specimen.

13. Promotes visualization of the sinuses.

14. Ensures the swab will be covered with the appropriate exudate.

15. Prevents contamination from normal nasal flora and erroneous culture results.

16. Prevents identification mistakes.

17. Reduces transmission of microorganisms.

18. Allows for access to the nasopharyngeal area.

continues

Collecting a Sputum Culture

19. Explain to the client that the specimen must be sputum, coughed up from the back of his throat or lungs.

19. Promotes client cooperation.

20. Have a sterile specimen cup ready for the sample and some tissue at hand.

20. The specimen must be collected in a sterile cup to prevent contamination.

21. Have the client take several deep breaths and then cough deeply (see Figure 1-14-8).

21. Helps to loosen secretions so the client will be able to provide a specimen.

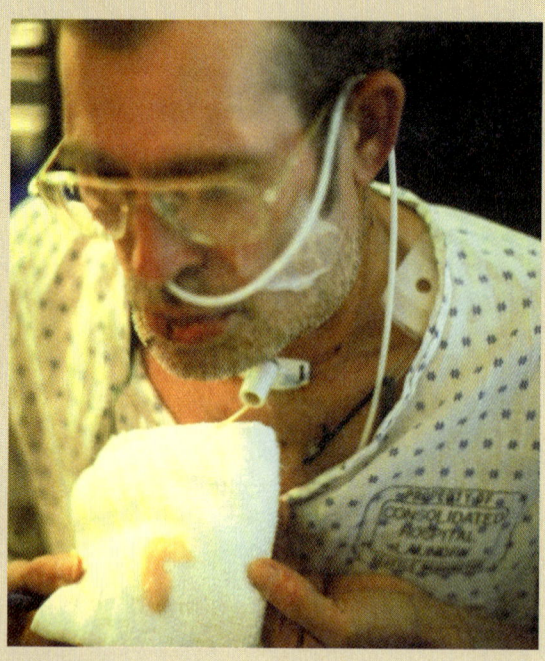

Figure 1-14-8 Have the client cough deeply.

22. Have the client expectorate the sputum into the sterile cup without touching the inside of the cup.

22. Prevents contamination of the specimen.

23. Place the lid on the specimen container without touching the inside of the lid or the container.

23. Prevents contamination of the specimen.

24. Provide the client with tissues and make him comfortable.

24. Promotes client comfort.

Alternative Sputum Collection Method
Generally used if the client is unable to expectorate an adequate sample

25. Obtain a sterile suction catheter and an inline sputum collection container.

25. Prevents contamination of the specimen.

SKILL 1-14 Collecting Nose, Throat, and Sputum Specimens

26. Provide the client with warm humidified air for about 20 minutes if it is not contraindicated by his condition.

27. Hook up the sputum collector to the suction tubing and a suction device (see Figure 1-14-9). Hook up the suction catheter to the sputum collector.

26. Helps to loosen secretions in the lungs.

27. Prepare the equipment prior to having the client cough.

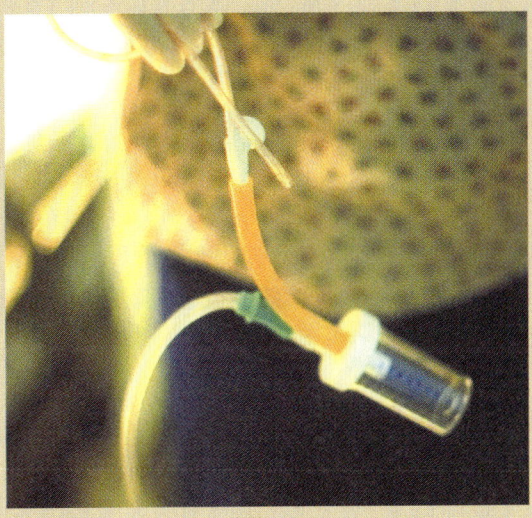

Figure 1-14-9 Sputum collector for use with suction.

28. If the client is able to cooperate, have him take several deep breaths and cough.

29. As the client is coughing up sputum, carefully insert the catheter either orally or nasopharyngeally into the back of the throat and suction the sputum into the specimen container.

30. Safely dispose of the suction catheter.

31. Close the specimen container.

32. Provide tissues or other measures for patient comfort.

33. Wash hands.

34. Label each specimen with the client's name.

35. Send the specimen to the laboratory.

28. Loosens the secretions and brings them up to the back of the throat.

29. Obtains a sterile specimen that is not contaminated with saliva.

30. Prevents the spread of microorganisms.

31. Prevents contamination of the specimen.

32. Promotes client comfort.

33. Reduces transmission of microorganisms.

34. Promotes the correct diagnosis for the client.

35. Provides the most accurate results.

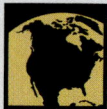

> ▶ **REAL WORLD ANECDOTES**
> When a respiratory syncytial virus (RSV) epidemic broke out in the city, school children were lined up to have throat cultures taken. Many of the children were frightened, and their parents were impatient. Three nurses were taking the cultures, and the child at the head of the line was supposed to go to the next available nurse. Danny was next in line and saw Nurse Prezbindowski. Danny was frightened, and his mother was angry about the long wait. Danny was crying, and his mother had to hold him and encourage him as the nurse took the throat culture. Danny's mother was obviously upset by the procedure and vented her frustrations to Nurse Prezbindowski. The culture was finally obtained, and Danny and his mother quickly left the room. After they left, Nurse Prezbindowski discovered that Danny's mother had not fully completed the laboratory form. She did not put an address or a phone number on the form. Nurse Prezbindowski was not able to contact Danny's mother to obtain the information, and without that information Danny's culture could not be processed by the lab. Danny's long wait and fearful cooperation was jeopardized by the missing information. Complete paperwork was required before the sample could be submitted to the lab. Before Danny and his mother left, the nurse should have reviewed the paperwork.

▶ EVALUATION

- An adequate specimen was obtained.
- The procedure was performed with a minimum of trauma to the patient.

▶ DOCUMENTATION

Nurses' Notes

- Record the date, time, and site from which the specimen was obtained.
- Note any bleeding or obvious trauma as a result of the procedure.
- Chart the description and time the specimen was collected. Note if the specimen is the first morning specimen, not pooled secretions.

▶ CRITICAL THINKING SKILL

Introduction

An accurate specimen is necessary so that appropriate treatment can be initiated.

Possible Scenario

Mr. Habakangus was admitted to the hospital with suspected pneumonia. His doctor had ordered a sputum specimen in order to definitely diagnose pneumonia and determine what microorganism was causing the infection. You bring Mr. Habakangus a sterile specimen cup and explain the procedure to him. Mr. Habakangus speaks very little English, but he seems to understand what you are asking him to do. He takes several deep breaths, coughs, and spits into the cup. The specimen is obviously saliva and you attempt to explain again that what is needed is sputum from his lungs. He tries to provide the needed specimen once more, but again he is able to provide only saliva.

Possible Outcome

You report to Mr. Habakangus' physician that you were unable to obtain a specimen. Without an accurate culture and sensitivity, his physician will have to prescribe a broad-spectrum antibiotic and hope it will work against the pneumonia. Mr. Habakangus may or may not get better quickly. His hospital stay and illness could be unnecessarily prolonged.

You reassure Mr. Habakangus and place a heated mist mask on him to help loosen the secretions. After about 15 minutes, you return with a sterile suction catheter, suction tubing, and an inline specimen container. You explain to Mr. Habakangus that you will try to suction the sputum from the back of his throat. You assure him that the procedure is a little unpleasant but not painful. Once again you instruct him to take several deep breaths and cough, but you ask him to cough with his mouth open so you can insert the suction catheter. When you use the catheter to suction his airway, the specimen in the cup is green and thick and appears to be sputum. You dispose of the catheter, cap the specimen cup, and comfort Mr. Habakangus. Because a sterile sputum specimen was obtained, the doctor will be able to pinpoint what organism is causing the pneumonia and how best to treat it.

Prevention

Educate the client regarding the importance of obtaining an actual sputum specimen and not saliva. Saliva has diagnostic value; sending an inadequate specimen only delays appropriate treatment of the client.

▶ VARIATIONS

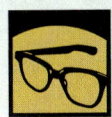

Geriatric Variation:
- Older clients may have difficulty tilting their head back due to osteoarthritis.

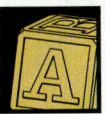

Pediatric Variations:
- Showing the tongue blade and penlight to a child before inserting them into the mouth may decrease anxiety.
- Ask the parent to help gently hold a child's head while obtaining a nose or throat culture.

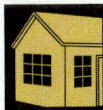

Home Care Variation:
- When obtaining a specimen that will not be sent to the lab right away, be sure to store it in a cool place to prevent growth.

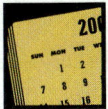

Long-Term-Care Variation:
- When obtaining a specimen that will not be sent to the lab right away, be sure to store it in a cool place to prevent growth.

▶ COMMON ERRORS

Possible Error:

The agitated, confused client moves his head while a nasal culture is being obtained, contaminating the specimen and causing bleeding.

Prevention:

Assess the client's ability to hold still during the procedure.

Stop the bleeding by applying pressure to the bridge of the nose. Use a new culture swab and ask for assistance from a coworker to help stabilize the client's head while obtaining the culture.

Possible Error:

The client gags on the tongue blade and contaminates the swab with his tongue.

Prevention:

Instruct the client on how to obtain a throat culture.

Remove the tongue blade and swab. Obtain a new culture swab. Ask the client to relax and take deep breaths. Depress the tongue blade on only the anterior half of the tongue. Swab the throat.

▶ **NURSING TIPS**

- Ask the parent or caregiver for assistance in obtaining the culture.
- Have the appropriate culture media available.
- Reassure the client of the short time of the procedure.
- Loosen the swab in the tube before having the client open his mouth for obtaining the throat culture.

▶ **SPECIAL CONSIDERATIONS**

- *Sputum specimens are best collected right after the client awakens, before ingesting anything by mouth (including fluids), and before brushing teeth or rinsing the mouth. If the client has eaten or brushed his teeth, rinse with water and wait from 15–30 minutes before collecting a throat specimen.*
- *It is essential to ensure an adequate specimen. Have the client use a deep cough to force out sputum. Nebulized saline solution may be necessary to facilitate adequate sputum production.*
- *If a specimen was collected and found unlabeled with the time collected, discard and obtain a new specimen.*
- *Copious amount of purulent sputum mixed with blood may be associated with bronchiectasis; pink sputum is suggestive of pulmonary edema fluid. Currant jelly sputum may be indicative of necrotizing pneumonia; putrid sputum, which is foul smelling, is found in lung abscesses.*
- *If the client is on antimicrobial therapy, specimen results will be of limited value due to suppression of microbials.*
- *Repeated sputum specimens may be of limited value in some conditions. For certain specimens, such as those for mycobacteria, 3 consecutive first morning specimens (not pooled) are optimal.*
- *If hemoptysis is present it is of diagnostic value. Chart the description and notify the appropriate staff.*
- *Sputum cytology may be used to identify certain cell types in cancer. A negative cytology result does not rule out disease.*

SKILL 1-15 Testing for Occult Blood with a Hemoccult Slide

Kathy Lilleby, RN and Gaylene Bouska Altman, RN, PhD

KEY TERMS

Feces
Gastrointestinal
Guaiac
Intestinal
Occult blood
Stool

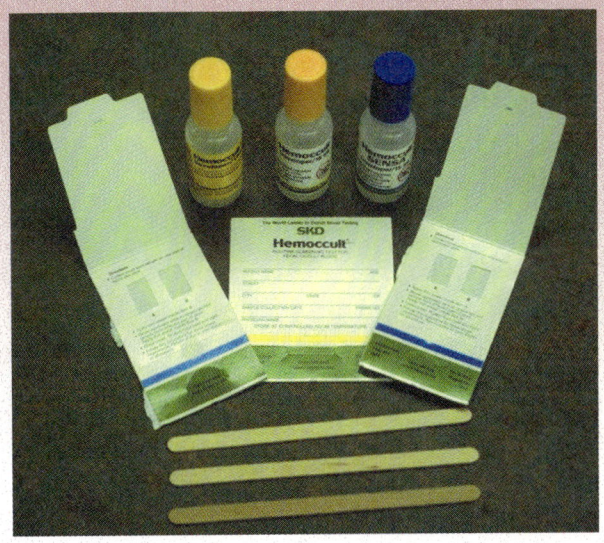

▶ OVERVIEW OF THE SKILL

Rectal examination and stool tests for occult blood are the best simple screening procedures for detecting a gastrointestinal (GI) tumor. The fecal occult blood test (FOBT), also known as the guaiac or guaiac-based test, detects microscopic amounts of blood in the stool. Usually this blood is *occult* (not grossly visible), although it may be observable. When blood is present in the stool, a color change is visualized by the use of hydrogen peroxidase on guaiac-impregnated paper. The test is useful in diagnosing gastric or intestinal irritation, GI bleed, upper GI ulcers, and colon cancer. When more than 50 cc of blood enters the feces from the upper GI tract, the stool becomes darker and is called *melena*.

Hemorrhoids, rectal fissures, or rectal trauma can lead to blood in the stool. Blood can also appear in the stool from cancers, ulcers, or ulcerative colitis. When the blood originates from the upper GI tract the stool is often black ("tarry"), whereas lower GI bleeding may still show unchanged blood and color the stool red. In the case of stool guaiac there is significant improvement in the detection rate when more than one specimen is obtained. This easy test requires only a small amount of stool, and the client can be instructed how to collect the specimen at home.

▶ ASSESSMENT

1. Assess the client's or family member's understanding of the need for this test **so the nurse can provide needed teaching.**
2. Assess the client's ability to cooperate with the procedure to collect the specimen **to maintain privacy while a sample is obtained.**
3. Assess the client's medical history for bleeding or GI disorders. **The nurse can initiate screening tests.**
4. Assess any medications the client receives that can cause GI bleeding, such as anticoagulants, steroids, or acetylsalicylic acid, **to help determine the need for the test, and/or the possible source of bleeding.**

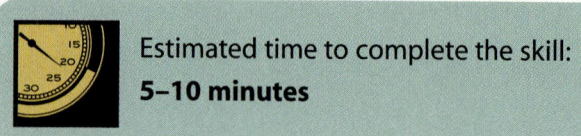

Estimated time to complete the skill: **5–10 minutes**

▶ DIAGNOSIS

- Constipation.
- Diarrhea.
- Deficient Knowledge, regarding the need and procedure of the test.

▶ PLANNING

Expected Outcomes:

1. The client will understand the purpose of the test.
2. The client will be able to collect the specimen, or allow the specimen to be collected.
3. The test for occult blood will be conducted properly and results will be recorded.

Equipment Needed (see Figure 1-15-1):

- Paper towel
- Disposable gloves
- Wooden applicator
- Occult blood test kit: Hemoccult slide and Hemoccult developing solution or Hematest tablets with guaiac-impregnated paper

▶ CLIENT EDUCATION NEEDED

1. The client should be taught the rationale for the stool test.

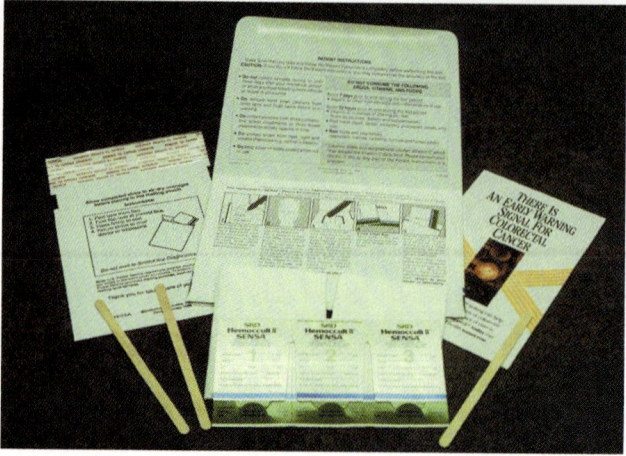

Figure 1-15-1 Hemoccult slide test kit to test for occult blood

2. The client should be instructed to avoid red meat for 24 hours before the test due to the possibility of producing a false-positive result.
3. Reassure the client that a simple positive test does not confirm a diagnosis of rectal bleeding or colorectal cancer. Three tests need to be done as well as further testing, such as a sigmoidoscopy.
4. Ask the client to list all medications he/she is taking in order to assess which ones he should not take before the Hemoccult test.
5. If the client is collecting the specimen, he/she should be instructed how to collect the specimen from two different areas of the stool.
6. The client should be told to keep the specimen free of urine and tissue.

▶ DELEGATION TIPS

The collection and testing of stool for occult blood may be delegated. Ancillary personnel should be instructed to report the presence of red blood in the stool immediately to the nurse. Positive results indicated on the hemoccult slide should be reported immediately to the nurse and recorded on the appropriate clinical record.

SKILL 1-15 Testing for Occult Blood with a Hemoccult Slide

IMPLEMENTATION—ACTION/RATIONALE

ACTION	RATIONALE
1. Wash hands and apply clean gloves.	1. Reduces transmission of microorganisms from fecal specimen to nurse.
2. Obtain a stool specimen from the client, commode, specimen cup, or bedpan.	2. Uncontaminated specimen will be in a dry container without urine, water, or tissue.
3. Obtain a small portion of feces with a wooden applicator.	3. Test can be performed on a small specimen.
4. Read and follow the manufacturer's instructions.	4. Ensures accurate results.

Perform Occult Blood Slide Test

5. Open the flap of the slide and smear a thin sample of feces on the paper in first box.	5. Guaiac-impregnated paper is sensitive to fecal blood.
6. Apply feces from a different area of the specimen to the second box.	6. Occult blood from the upper GI tract is not always equally dispersed throughout the stool.
7. Close the slide cover and turn to the reverse side. Open the flap and apply two drops of developing solution on each sample box and on each control box according to the manufacturer's instructions (see Figure 1-15-2).	7. Developing solution penetrates the fecal specimen through the paper.
8. Note color change after 60 seconds or according to manufacturer's instructions.	8. Bluish color indicates the presence of occult blood. Control box color can be used for comparison. No change in color is negative.
9. Dispose of slide and applicator wrapped in a paper towel in the proper receptacle. Remove gloves and wash hands.	9. Reduces transfer of microorganisms.

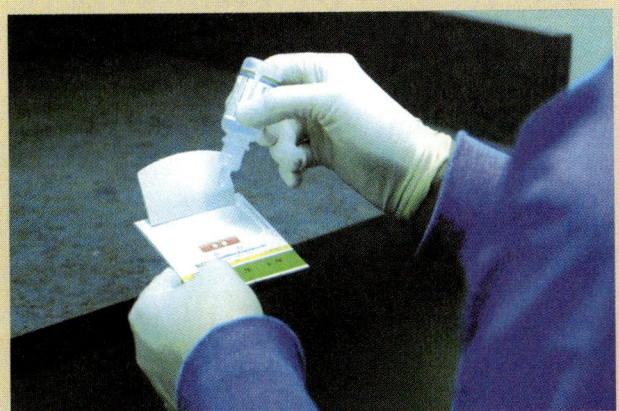

Figure 1-15-2 Apply the developing solution to the slide.

continues

Perform Hematest continued

10. Apply a small amount of feces on guaiac-impregnated paper.	10. Guaiac-impregnated paper is sensitive to fecal blood.
11. Place a Hematest tablet on top of the stool specimen.	11. Tablet contains solid form of developing solution.
12. Apply 2–3 drops of tap water to the tablet.	12. Tap water dissolves tablet, which releases solution over the specimen and paper.
13. Note color change after 2 minutes.	13. Bluish color indicates the presence of occult blood. Results after 2 minutes may be false.
14. Dispose of tablet, paper, and applicator wrapped in a paper towel in the proper receptacle.	14. Reduces transmission of microorganisms.
15. Remove gloves and wash hands.	15. Reduces transmission of microorganisms.

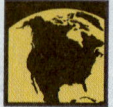

▶ REAL WORLD ANECDOTES

Martha had a family history of colorectal cancer so her physician recommended yearly screening for occult blood. The nurse taught her how to collect the specimen and how to apply a small sample of the stool onto the guaiac paper in the first box. Martha then showed the nurse how she would take a sample from another part of the stool and apply it to the second box. Satisfied with the return demonstration, the nurse gave Martha test kits for three days. The nurse told Martha to bring the kits to the office when she had completed them. The nurse would develop the test and tell her the results.

▶ EVALUATION

- Note presence or absence of color change in the guaiac paper.
- Note color, character, and consistency of stool.
- Ask the client to explain the rationale and procedure for the stool test.

▶ DOCUMENTATION

Nurses' Notes

- Record the date and time the collection was obtained and the test performed.
- Record the results of the test.
- Record the color, character, and consistency of the stool.
- Record when the results of the test were reported to the physician or qualified practitioner.

▶ CRITICAL THINKING SKILL

Introduction

There are several causes for a false-positive occult blood test. One is eating red meat or citrus fruit; another is taking medications, such as iron preparations, aspirin, anticoagulants, ascorbic acid, steroids, or indomethicin. Hemorrhoids can cause bleeding and may be misinterpreted as upper or lower GI bleeding.

Possible Scenario

A client noticed small flecks of blood in his stool. He was instructed to collect a stool sample and apply it to an occult blood kit. When the nurse developed it, the results were strongly positive.

Possible Outcome

The nurse reviewed the client's history and found that he had received treatment for hemorrhoids in the past. The client also admitted he had failed to stop taking his daily aspirin prescribed by his cardiologist.

Prevention

A careful health assessment would have revealed these two common reasons for blood in the stool—hemorrhoids and taking aspirin.

SKILL 1-15 Testing for Occult Blood with a Hemoccult Slide

▶ VARIATIONS

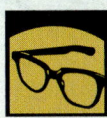
Geriatric Variation:
- Some clients will need to bring the entire stool sample in a plastic specimen container if they are unable to use the occult blood test kit.

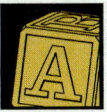
Pediatric Variations:
- Children may not be able to produce a specimen at a given time. Parents may need to assist them at home.
- Small children may be curious about what is done to the sample. They should be allowed to watch the test being done.

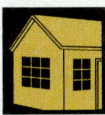
Home Care Variation:
- If the specimen is collected at home, the client should be instructed how to store it before it is brought to the laboratory.

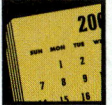
Long-Term-Care Variation:
- Review correct testing procedures with staff who may not be familiar with the test. If the test must be repeated periodically, encourage the client to be as independent as possible collecting the sample.

▶ COMMON ERRORS

Possible Error:
The stool becomes contaminated with urine.

Prevention:
Use a plastic insert in the toilet to facilitate collection of the stool (see Figure 1-15-3).

Discard the stool and wait for the next opportunity to collect a stool sample.

Possible Error:
The nurse opens the developing flap to apply the smear of stool.

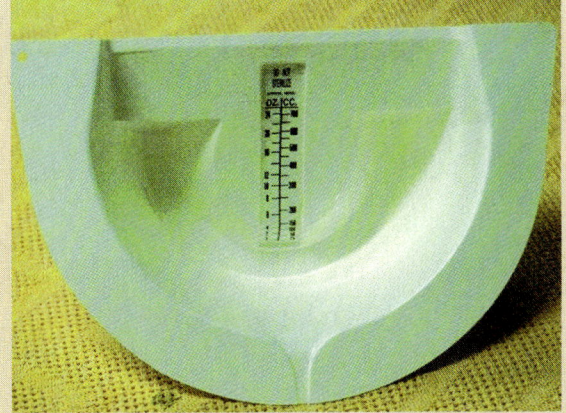
Figure 1-15-3 Use a graduated specimen container to collect a stool sample.

Prevention:
Read the directions on the flap to choose the correct side to apply the sample.

Discard the Hemoccult slide and use a new one to apply the stool to the correct side. Proceed with the development of the test.

▶ NURSING TIPS

- Using a plastic insert in the toilet may facilitate obtaining a stool specimen.
- Occult blood should be tested regardless of the character or color of the stool, i.e., Bismuth (Pepto Bismol) produces black stool in the absence of bleeding. Black or tarry stools do not exclude a diagnosis of GI bleeding. Red, black, or melena stool may be an indication of GI bleeding.
- Check the lot number and brand name to ensure efficacy of the developing solution or slide. Mixing brand names can diminish the reliability of the reaction.
- Stool specimens should be tested within 48 hours after collection.

▶ SPECIAL CONSIDERATIONS

- *Stool tested for occult blood may have positive results up to 14 days after a single, major episode of upper GI bleeding.*
- *False positive results are related to ingestion of red fruits and meats, methylene blue, chlorophyll, iodide, cupric sulfate, and bromide preparations.*
- *False negative results are rare but may be caused by bile or from ingestion of magnesium-containing antacids or ascorbic acid.*
- *A hemoccult test may be unreliable to evaluate gastric contents for occult blood.*
- *In newborns, maternal blood that is swallowed may cause bloody stools. (The Apt test may demonstrate that it is maternal in origin.)*

Index

A

Abdomen, 19-20
Abdominal breathing, 15, 19
Accessory muscles, 15
Achilles' reflexes, 22
Achilles' tendon, 22
Activities of daily living (ADLs), 25
Airways, 52-7
Alcohol abuse, 28
Alcohol swabs, 44, 119
Allen test, 45
Ancillary personnel
    blood glucose testing, 122
    blood pressure measurement, 59
    educational efforts, 91
    educational role, 82
    input and output measurements, 76
    occult blood testing, 138
    radial pulse assessment, 45
    respiratory rate measurement, 54
    skin punctures, 115
    specimen collection, 100, 129
    temperature measurement, 30
    urine testing, 107
    weighing clients, 68
Ankles, assessment, 22
Anterior cervical chain lymph nodes, 9
Anthropometric measurements, 7
Anticoagulants, 113
Antipyretics, 40
Anus, 21
Anxiety, 7
Apical pulses
    assessment, 16, 45, 47-8
    infants, 49
    older clients, 49
Apnea, 53
Appearance, general, 3, 7
Arteriovenous shunts, 65
Aspirin, 113
Assessment, definition, 2
Assessment forms, 4
Athletes, respiratory rates, 57
Atrial fibrillation, 16
Audio testing equipment, 5
Auscultation
    apical pulses, 47-8
    blood pressure measurement, 58, 60-3
    heart sounds, 16-19, 18
    lungs, 14, 16
    in physical assessment, 3
    pulses, 43
    rhonchi, 28
Axillary lymph nodes, 13

B

Babinski reflex, 23
Back, assessment, 14
Balance scales, 69
Barrel chest, 15
Bedpans, 76
Biceps reflex, 13
Blood collection, 116
Blood glucose, 120-7
Blood pressure, 7, 58-66
Blood pressure cuffs, 5, 60-3
Body temperature
    assessment of, 29-42
    axillary measurement, 37-8
    comparison of methods, 41
    delegation, 30
    normal ranges, 41
    oral, 31-2, 34-6
    rectal measurement, 36-7
    skin, 2
    skin measurement, 38
    Tempa-Dot measurement, 33-4
    tympanic measurement, 33
Body weight
    breast size and, 81
    importance, 67
    intake and output measurements, 74-80
    loss, 107
    measurement, 67-73
Bowel sounds, 97
Brachial arteries, 60-3
Brachial pulses, 13, 45
Brachioradialis reflex, 13
Bradypnea, 52
Breast cancer, 81
Breasts
    developmental stages, 89
    examination, 13, 28
    male, 81
    pain, 89
    postmenopausal, 81
    self-examination, 5, 81-9
Bucal mucosa, 12

C

Calibration, scales, 69
Capillaries, 114, 120
Carbon dioxide, 66
Cardiac arrest, 45
Cardiovascular system, 16-19
Carotid pulses, 12, 45, 49, 50
Centigrade, 41
Cerebellar status, 24
Cervical spine, 13, 14
Charts, 4
Checklists, 27
Chest
    anterior, 15
    AP measurement, 28
    examination, 13
    movement, 52
Cheyne-Stokes respirations, 15, 53
Children. see also Infants; Newborns
    blood pressures, 66
    electrolyte imbalances, 79
    heart sounds, 17
    lymph nodes, 8
    parents as witnesses, 88
    respiratory rates, 55
Circulation, 45, 50, 66
Clean-catch specimen, 99
Clean-voided specimens, 99
Clients education, 5, 6
Clinistix, 106
Coffee grounds, 4
Colostrum, 87
Communications
    geriatric clients, 26
    pediatric clients, 26-7
    supportive environment for, 6
Confidentiality, 5
Conjunctivae, 10
Contractures, 25
Corneal touch reflex, 10, 23
Corneas, 10
Cortical sensations, 23
Cotton balls, 4
Cotton swabs, 4, 129
Coughing techniques, 54
Coughs, 15
Cranial nerves, 10, 11, 12, 23-4
Cremasteric reflex, 21, 90, 93
Culture medium, 129
Currant jelly sputum, 136
Cyanosis, 15, 53

D

Dates, documentation, 25
Deep-breathing, 54
Delegation
    blood glucose testing, 122
    blood pressure measurement, 59
    educational efforts, 91
    input and output measurements, 76
    occult blood testing, 138
    radial pulse assessment, 45
    respiratory rate measurement, 54
    skin punctures, 115
    specimen collection, 100, 129

urine testing, 107
weighing clients, 68
Denver Developmental Screening Kit, 5
Diabetes, 53, 120-7
Diapers, 79, 80, 112
Diaphragm, 20, 52
Diarrhea, 79
Diastix, 106
Diastolic blood pressure, 62
Diastolic gallop, 17
Diffusion, definition, 66
Dipsticks, 106, 110-11
Distress, signs of, 7
Documentation
    assessment forms, 4
    blood glucose testing, 124-5
    blood pressures, 64
    body temperature, 30
    breast examination, 86
    client charts, 25
    confidentiality, 5
    fluid intake and output, 76, 78
    height, 4
    I/O flow sheets, 80
    male genital examination, 96
    occult blood testing, 140
    pulses, 49
    respiratory rates, 56
    skin punctures, 118
    specimen collection, 103, 134
    urine test results, 111
    vital signs flow sheet, 38
    weight, 4, 72
Domestic violence, 28
Doppler ultrasonography, 5, 43-4, 50, 66
Dorsalis pedis pulses, 22, 45, 58
Drape sheets, 4
Drug abuse, 28
Dullness, description, 2
Dyspnea, 53

E

Earlobes, 114
Ears, 11
Education of clients
    during assessment, 5
    blood glucose testing, 122
    blood pressure measurement, 59
    capillary puncture, 114-15
    intake and output issues, 75
    measuring body temperature, 30
    occult blood testing, 138
    pulse rates, 44
    self-examination, 5, 50, 82
    sexually-transmitted diseases, 5
    specimen collection, 100, 129
    urinary hygiene, 5
    weight measurement, 68
Elbows, 13
Electrolyte imbalances, 79
Electronic scales, 69
Emesis basins, 129
Emesis volume, 79
Exteroceptive sensations, 23
Environment, assessment of, 3
Equilibrium, 23
Equipment
    blood glucose testing, 121
    blood pressure measurement, 59
    breast self-examinations, 82
    capillary puncture, 114
    intake and output measurement, 75
    male genital examination, 91
    measuring body temperature, 30
    occult blood testing, 138
    organization, 6
    pediatric clients and, 26-7
    physical assessment, 4-5
    specimen collection, 100, 128-9
    urine testing, 107
Erb's point, 17
Eupnea, 52
Exercise, 113
Extraocular mobility, 10, 23
Extremities, lower, 3, 21-2, 45
Eye covers, 5
Eyes, assessment, 10-11

F

Face, assessment, 8-9
Facial expressions, 7, 23
Fahrenheit, 41
Family medical history, 82, 98
Fatigue, 107
Feces, 137
Feet, 22, 24
Femoral hernia, 94
Femoral pulses, 20, 45
Fetal heart rate, 50
Fibrocystic breast disease, 89
Fingernails, 4
Fingers, 13
Fingertips, 114, 127
Flashlights, 5
Flatness, description, 2
Fluid balance, 74, 75
Fluid retention, 74
Fluid volume, 67
Foley drainage bags, 77
Follow-up care, 6
Fontanelles, 8
Fremitus, 14, 15, 16
Frenula, 12

G

Gag reflex, 12, 23
Gait assessment, 7, 21, 25
Gallant reflex, 22
Gas exchange, 52-7, 66
Gastric air bubble, 20
Gastroenteritis, 79
Genitalia, male, 90-8
Geriatric variations
    blood glucose testing, 126
    blood pressure measurements, 64
    breast examinations, 87
    electrolyte imbalances, 79
    intake output balance, 79
    male genital examination, 97
    occult blood testing, 141
    physical assessment, 26
    pulse taking, 49
    respiratory rate assessment, 56
    skin punctures, 118
    specimen collection, 104, 135
    temperature measurement, 39
    urine testing, 112
    weighing clients, 72
Glans penis, 92
Gloves, 5, 30, 31, 44, 129
Glucose
    blood levels, 120-7
    dipstick tests, 110-11
    urine testing, 106
Glucose meters, 120
Goiter, 12
Goniometer, 5
Gowns, 4, 5
Graphesthesia, 23
Grip, assessment, 13
Grooming, assessment, 7
Guaiac card, 5, 137, 139
Guarding, 7
Gums, assessment, 12
Gynecomastia, 89

H

Hair, 7-8. see also Pubic hair
Hands, assessment, 13
Handwashing, 5, 6, 31
Hard palate, 12
Head, assessment, 8
Headlamps, 5
Health assessment, 2
Hearing, 11, 23
Heart
    assessment, 16-19
    mnemonic, 28
    rates, 7
    rhythms, 7
    sounds, 18
    valve mnemonic, 28
Heel sticks, 118, 126
Height, 4
Hematest, 138
Hemoccult slides, 137-42
Hemoptysis, 136
Hemorrhoids, 137
Hernias, 90-8, 94, 97
Herpetic lesions, 29
Hips, assessment, 22
Hirschberg's corneal light reflex, 10
Home care variations
    blood glucose testing, 126
    blood pressure measurement, 65
    breast examination, 87
    intake output balance, 79
    male genital examination, 97
    occult blood testing, 141
    physical assessment, 27
    pulse taking, 50
    respiratory rate assessment, 56
    skin punctures, 118
    specimen collection, 104, 135
    temperature measurement, 39
    urine testing, 112
    weighing clients, 72
Hydroceles, 21, 97
Hygiene, assessment, 7
Hyperpnea, 15, 52
Hyperresonance, 2
Hypertension, 58

INDEX

Hyperventilation, 52
Hypotension, 58
Hypothermia, 29
Hypoventilation, 52
Hyspnea, 15

I

I/O flow sheets, 80
Ice chips, 80
Identification bands, 115
Iliac crests, 21
Incontinence, 97
Infants. see also Children; Newborns
    abdominal breathing, 15, 19
    blood pressure measurement, 66
    brachial pulses, 45
    capillary punctures, 114
    carotid pulses, 45
    cremasteric reflex, 21
    fluid imbalance, 79
    hearing acuity tests, 11
    hip click, 22
    nipple discharge, 87
    PMI in, 49
    radial pulse, 49
    reflexes, 22-3
    respiratory rates, 55
    temporal pulses, 45
Infection control
    alcohol swabs, 44
    body fluid outputs, 80
    electronic thermometers, 31
    gloves, 31, 44
    handwashing, 6
    herpetic lesions, 29
    lancets, 127
    output measurement, 77-8
    scales, 69, 71
Infections, fevers and, 29
Inguinal hernias, 94
Inspection, 2
Intake, measuring, 74-80
Introductions, 5
IPPA (inspection, palpation, percussion, auscultation), 2
Irises, assessment, 10

J

Joints, lower extremities, 22
Jugular vein distention (JVD), 19

K

Ketoacidosis, 53
Ketones, 106, 107, 110-11
Knees, assessment, 22
Korotkoff sounds, 62, 66
Kussmaul's respirations, 53
Kyphosis, 25

L

Labstix, 106
Lactation, 87
Lancets, 114, 116, 127
Landau reflex, 22

Legal issues, self-protection, 88
Lips, 12, 15
Lithotomy position, 20
Liver, palpation, 28
Long-term care variations
    blood glucose testing, 126
    blood pressure measurement, 65
    breast examinations, 87
    intake output balance, 79
    male genital examination, 97
    occult blood testing, 141
    physical assessment, 27
    pulse taking, 50
    respiratory rate assessment, 56
    skin punctures, 118
    specimen collection, 104, 135
    temperature measurement, 39
    urine testing, 112
    weighing clients, 72
Lordsis, 25
Lubricants, 5, 30
Lungs, 14, 136
Lymph nodes
    assessment, 8-9
    axillary, 13, 85
    epitrochlear, 13
    head and neck, 9
    infraclavicular, 84
    inguinal, 20, 21
    subclavian, 84
    supraventricular, 84

M

Magnifying glasses, 5
Mammograms, 81
Mannerisms, assessment, 7
Masks, 5
Mastectomies, 66
Mastoid, assessment, 11
Measuring tapes, 5
Medical conditions, assessment, 3
Medical history, 3, 6, 44, 83
Melena, 137
Menstrual blood, 104, 107
Mental status assessment, 24
Mercury toxicity, 42
Microhematocrit tubes, 114
Micropipettes, 114
Midstream specimens, 99
Mini-mental status examination, 5
Mitral stenosis, 17
Mitral valve, 17
Mitral valve prolapse, 17
Mnemonics, 28
Mood, assessment, 7
Moro reflex, 22
Motor movements, 7
Mouth, assessment, 12
Multistix, 106
Murmurs, pulmonic, 17
Musculoskeletal examination, 21-2
Mycobacteria, 136

N

Nails, assessment, 7-8
Nasal cultures, 131
Nasal speculum, 5

Nasopharyngeal cultures, 131
Neck, assessment, 12
Neurological assessment, 3, 22-5
Neurological kits, 5
Neuromuscular examination, upper, 13
Newborns
    capillary punctures, 114, 118
    fontanelles, 8
    occult blood testing, 142
    sutures, 8
Nipples, 83, 88
Nose, 12, 128-36
Nutritional status
    assessment, 7
    measuring intake and output, 74-80
    urine test results and, 113
    weight and, 67-73
Nystagmus, 10

O

Obesity, 50
Observation, inspection and, 2
Occipital lymph nodes, 9
Occult blood
    dipstick tests, 110-11
    testing for, 137-42
    urine testing, 106
Odors, 7, 12, 23
Ophthalmoscopes, 4
Oral temperature, 29
Orange extract, 4
Orthostatic hypotension, 58
Ortolani's sign, 22
Osler's sign, 64
Osteoarthritis, 21
Otoscopes, 4, 5, 11
Output, measuring, 74-80
Oxygen exchange, 66

P

Palmer grasp reflex, 22
Palpation
    blood pressure measurement, 58
    breast, 84
    carotid pulses, 12
    hernias, 94
    lips, 12
    liver, 28
    lymph nodes, 9-10
    neck, 12
    in physical assessment, 2
    precordium, 16
    prostate gland, 95
    pulses, 43
    radial pulse, 46-7
    skin, 8
    temporal pulses, 12
Paradoxic pulse, 66
Paravertebral muscle spasms, 21
Patellar reflexes, 22
Pectus carinatum, 15
Pectus excavatum, 15
Pedal pulses, 45, 50
Pediatric variations
    blood glucose testing, 126
    blood pressure measurement, 65
    breast examinations, 87

intake output balance, 79
male genital examination, 97
occult blood testing, 141
physical assessment, 26-7
pulse taking, 49-50
respiratory rate assessment, 56
skin punctures, 118
specimen collection, 104, 135
temperature measurement, 39
urine testing, 112
weighing clients, 72
Penis, 21, 91-2
Penlights, 4, 129
Pens, 4, 5
Percussion, 2, 14, 15, 20
PH, urine, 107
Phoria, 10
Physical assessments
equipment, 4-5
geriatric variations, 26
home care variations, 27
long-term care variations, 27
measurements, 7
pediatric variations, 26-7
systemic approach, 2-28
Plantar grasp reflex, 22
Pleura, 52
Pneumonia, 136
Polydypsia, 107
Polyphagia, 107
Polyuria, 107
Popliteal pulses, 22, 45
Postauricular lymph nodes, 9
Posterior cervical chain lymph nodes, 10
Posterior tibial pulses, 22, 45
Posture, 7, 21, 24
Preauricular lymph nodes, 9
Precordium, palpation, 16
Pregnancy variations, 87
Privacy
long-term care setting, 27
patient comfort and, 6
during physical assessment, 4
specimen collection, 100
temperature measurement and, 31
Problem-solving strategies, 3
Propioceptive sensations, 23
Prostate gland, 90, 95
Prostate-specific antigen (PSA), 98
Proteinuria, 113
Psychiatric symptoms, 25
Puberty, 81, 87
Pubic hair, 21, 90, 92, 97
Pulse points, 45
Pulses. see also Specific pulse points
assessment of, 43-51
duration of monitoring efforts, 50
measuring volume, 49
Pulus paradoxus, 66
Pupils, 10, 23
Pyrexia, 29, 79
Pyrogens, 29

R

Radial arteries, 58
Radial pulses
assessment, 13, 16, 45, 46-7
delegation of assessment, 45
infants, 49

Range of motion (ROM), 13, 21, 22
Rapid alternating hand movement (RAHM) test, 24
Receptiveness, assessment of, 3
Rectal examinations, 90-8, 94-6, 137
Rectal fissures, 137
Rectus abdominus muscles, 19
Reflex hammers, 4, 5
Reflexes
abdominal, 20
Achilles', 22
Babinski, 23
biceps, 13
brachioradialis, 13
corneal touch, 10
cremasteric, 21, 90, 93
gag, 12, 23
Gallant, 22
Hirschberg's, 10
infantile, 22-3
Landau, 22
moro, 22
neurological examination, 22-3
palmer grasp, 22
patellar, 22
plantar grasp, 22
rooting, 22
stepping, 22
suck, 22
tonic neck, 22
triceps, 13
Refractometers, 106, 108, 109
Regulation of ventilation, 66
Resonance, 2
Resources, assessment, 3
Respirations
assessment, 15, 52-7
auscultation, 14
measurement, 7
normal rates, 52
patterns, 15, 53
rates in athletes, 57
Rhinne tests, 11, 23
Romberg tests, 24
Rhonchi, 28
Rooting reflex, 22

S

Salivary gland assessment, 12
Scales, 68, 73
Sclera, 10
Scoliosis, 21, 25
Scrotum, 21, 93-4
Self-examinations
breast, 81-9
teaching of, 5
testicular, 97
Seminal vesicles, 90, 96
Sensation, assessment, 23
Senses, assessment, 23
Sexual maturity
assessment, 21
female breast development, 89
male, 90
male genital examination, 97
Tanner stages, 13
Sexually-transmitted diseases, 5
Sharp items, 4
Sharps disposal, 117

Shock, 45
Shortness of breath (SOB), 15
Shoulders, 13, 24
Sighing, 52
Signatures, 25
Skin
assessment, 7-8
back, 14
elderly clients, 118
lower extremities, 22
palpation, 2
puncture of, 114-19, 120-7
self-examination, 5
Slides, 5
Sling scales, 70-1
Smegma, 92
Soft palate, 12
Specific gravity, 106, 108-10
Specimen collection
capillary blood, 116
identification, 115
nasal swabs, 128-36
sputum, 128-36
throat cultures, 128-36
urine, 99-105
Specimen cups, 5, 76, 100, 129
Speech, assessment, 7
Sphygmomanometers, 5, 58
Splinting positions, 15
Sputum, 128-36, 132-3
Standing balances, 68
Standing electronic scales, 68
Standing scales, 69
Starvation, 113
Stepping reflex, 22
Stereognosis, 23
Sterile swabs, 129
Sternocleidomastoid muscles, 24
Stethoscopes
apical pulses, 47-8
monitoring pulses, 44
pulses, 43
types, 5
use, 58
warming, 50
Stool, 137, 141
Strength testing, 13, 23
Stress, 28
Stridor, 15
Submandibular lymph nodes, 9
Submental lymph nodes, 9
Suck reflex, 22
Supernumerary nipples, 83
Supraclavicular lymph nodes, 10
Sutures, newborns, 8
Swallowing, 12, 23
Systolic blood pressure, 62

T

Tachypnea, 15, 52
Tanner stages, 13, 21, 90, 92, 97
Taste tests, 12
Teeth, assessment, 12
Temperature. see body temperature
Temporal pulses, 12, 45, 49
Test tapes, 106, 120
Test tubes, 5
Testicles, 5, 21, 90
Testicular torsion, 93, 98

Thermometers
    axillary measurement, 37-8
    comparison of methods, 41
    disposable chemical strip, 38
    electronic, 31-2
    oral, 34-6
    rectal, 34, 36-7
    Tempa-Dot, 33-4
    types, 5, 30
Thoracic spine, 14
Thorax, 15-16
Throat, 12, 128-36
Throat cultures, 130-1
Thyroid gland, 12, 14
Times, documentation, 25
Tongue, 12, 24
Tongue depressors, 4, 5, 129
Tonic neck reflex, 22
Tonsillar lymph nodes, 10
Toothbrushes, 5
Touch, assessment, 23
Trachea, assessment, 12
Transilluminators, 5
Transport, 66
Trapezius muscles, 24

Tremors, 49
Triceps reflex, 13
Tricuspid valve, 17
Tripod positions, 15
Tropia, 10
Tuning forks, 4
Tympanic membrane, 11, 33
Tympany, 2

U

Ulnar pulses, 45
Understanding, assessment, 3
Unistiks, 116
Urethral meatus, 21, 92
Urinary tract infections, 104
Urine
    output fluid volume, 75
    retention, 97
    specimen collection, 99-105
    specimen testing, 106-13
Urinometers, 106, 109-10
Uristix, 106
Uvula, 12, 28

V

Ventilation, definition, 66
Vision charts, 5, 11
Visual acuity, 11, 23
Visual fields, 11
Vital signs
    baseline data, 30-1
    blood pressures, 64
    measurement, 7
    respiratory rates, 56
Voice/whisper test, 11

W

Watch-tick test, 11
Watches, 5, 44, 54
Water, drinking, 5
Weber test, 11, 23
Weight, (see body weight), 67
Wood's lamp, 5
Wrists, assessment, 13